W9-BRV-876

The Hot Guide to Safer Sex

"What could be better than a smart responsible student of sexuality putting sex in the most important context today: safer sex. In a bright and reader-friendly tone, Yvonne K. Fulbright tells peers what they need to know to be healthy and prudent, while still being happy and passionate, in intimate relationships."

DR. JUDY KURIANSKY, Ph.D., Clinical Psychology
Adjunct Professor of Psychology
Columbia University Teachers College
Author, *The Complete Idiot's Guide to Dating* and
Generation Sex: America's Hottest Sex Therapist Answers the Hottest Questions about Sex

DEDICATION:

For my brother,

Xavier Þór Fulbright

Þú ert besti bróðirinn

í öllum heiminum!

ORDERING

Trade bookstores in the U.S. and Canada please contact:

Publishers Group West
1700 Fourth Street, Berkeley CA 94710
Phone: (800) 788-3123   Fax: (510) 528-3444

Hunter House books are available at bulk discounts for textbook course adoptions; to qualifying community, health-care, and government organizations; and for special promotions and fund-raising. For details please contact:

Special Sales Department
Hunter House Inc., PO Box 2914, Alameda CA 94501-0914
Phone: (510) 865-5282   Fax: (510) 865-4295
E-mail: sales@hunterhouse.com

Individuals can order our books from most bookstores, by calling **(800) 266-5592**, or from our website at **www.hunterhouse.com**

The Hot Guide
to
Safer Sex

Yvonne K. Fulbright, M.S.Ed. *

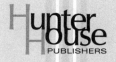

Hunter House
PUBLISHERS

Copyright © 2003 by Yvonne Fulbright

All rights reserved. No part of this publication may be reproduced or transmitted in any form or by any means, electronic or mechanical, including photocopying and recording, or introduced into any information storage and retrieval system without the written permission of the copyright owner and the publisher of this book. Brief quotations may be used in reviews prepared for inclusion in a magazine, newspaper, or for broadcast. For further information please contact:

Hunter House Inc., Publishers
PO Box 2914
Alameda CA 94501-0914

LIBRARY OF CONGRESS CATALOGING-IN-PUBLICATION DATA
Fulbright, Yvonne K.
  The hot guide to safer sex / Yvonne K. Fulbright.– 1st ed.
      p. cm.
Includes index.
  ISBN 0-89793-408-3 (hardcover) – ISBN 0-89793-407-5 (pbk)
  1. Sex instruction–Popular works. 2. Sex–Popular works. I. Title.
  HQ31.F85 2003
  613.9'6–dc21   2003005539

PROJECT CREDITS
Photographer: Donna Alberico
Illustrator: Lisa Kroin
Cover Design: Brian Dittmar Graphic Design
Book Production: Hunter House
Developmental Editor: Kelley Blewster
Copy Editor: Rachel E. Bernstein
Proofreader: John David Marion
Indexer: Deanna Butler
Acquisitions Editor: Jeanne Brondino
Editor: Alexandra Mummery
Publicity Coordinators: Earlita K. Chenault & Lisa E. Lee
Sales & Marketing Coordinator: Jo Anne Retzlaff
Customer Service Manager: Christina Sverdrup
Order Fulfillment: Lakdhon Lama
Administrator: Theresa Nelson
Computer Support: Peter Eichelberger
Publisher: Kiran S. Rana

Printed and bound by Bang Printing, Brainerd, Minnesota

Manufactured in the United States of America

9 8 7 6 5 4 3 2 1   First Edition   03 04 05 06 07

Contents

* Important Note *

THE MATERIAL IN THIS BOOK IS INTENDED TO
PROVIDE A REVIEW OF RESOURCES AND
INFORMATION RELATED TO SAFER SEX. EVERY
EFFORT HAS BEEN MADE TO PROVIDE ACCU-
RATE AND DEPENDABLE INFORMATION. WE
BELIEVE THAT THE SENSUALITY ADVICE GIVEN
IN THIS BOOK POSES NO RISK TO ANY
HEALTHY PERSON. HOWEVER, IF YOU HAVE
ANY SEXUALLY TRANSMITTED DISEASES, WE
RECOMMEND CONSULTING YOUR DOCTOR
BEFORE USING THIS BOOK.

THE AUTHOR, EDITORS, AND PUBLISHERS
CANNOT BE HELD RESPONSIBLE FOR ANY
ERROR, OMISSION, PROFESSIONAL DISAGREE-
MENT OR OUTDATED MATERIAL AND ARE
NOT LIABLE FOR ANY DAMAGE, INJURY, OR
OTHER ADVERSE OUTCOME OF APPLYING ANY
OF THE INFORMATION RESOURCES IN THIS
BOOK. IF YOU HAVE QUESTIONS CONCERN-
ING THE APPLICATION OF THE INFORMATION
DESCRIBED IN THIS BOOK, CONSULT A
QUALIFIED PROFESSIONAL.

Acknowledgments

This book would not have its depth or its unique flavor without the contributions of the many people who let me dig into their personal lives for quotes. Though I cannot list their names, I want to sincerely thank everyone who spilled their hearts and souls, enhancing this book with some of their deepest confessions. I am eternally grateful to all of them for their honesty, openness, and trust.

My deepest thanks to all of the wonderful people in my life who have not only been extremely supportive of this book project and my "sexpert" pursuits, but who have also made me the sexuality educator I am today: my parents, Charles G. Fulbright and Ósk Lárusdóttir Fulbright, my brother, Xavier Þór Fulbright, Dr. Konstance McCaffree, Dr. William Stayton, Dr. Andrew Behrendt, and Dr. Peter Kuriloff. I would also like to give mention and many thanks to my incredible friends and colleagues, who gave me great feedback on some of the chapters as I was plugging through this book: Rick Barth, Heather Behar, Marci Fields, Tiffany J. Franklin, Dr. Eric J. Hodgson, Christy Wetzel Kiely, Emily Kohnke, Megan Mead, Dr. Erika I. Pluhar, and Dr. Beverly Whipple. Merci beaucoup, too, for the support of everyone on my e-mail listserv for all of their suggestions, and to my sexpert endeavor cheerleaders: Dr. Simon Ahtaridis, Bianca Angelino, Dr. Edward L. Brown, Lauren Bryson, Fikre Deneke, Gunnlaugur Petur Erlendsson, Mia Kaminsky, Mr. Leon B. Kassman, Christopher Klimek, Brian S. Lerner, Luke F. Leubuscher, Nate Manifold, Brian McEntire, Michael McKenna, Fadi Nazzal, Alissa Nickey, Dr. Rian Podein, Michelle Radz, Dr. Jon Rittenberger, Betsy Schechter, Pam Schechter, Dr. Alyson Taub, Dr. Mitchell Tepper, Christian Thrasher, Thomas R. Turner, and Dr. S. Alexander Weinstock. You guys are the bomb!

Finally, a special thanks to my cousin, Eydís K. Sveinbjarnardóttir, for nurturing the "you should be a sexpert" seed in me when I was fifteen; to Merle Ginsberg, the entertainment editor of *W* magazine, for making that phone call in January of 1999, encouraging me to write a book; to my wonderful photographer, Donna Alberico, who was a dream to work with; to all of the beautiful models who bared all; to my super illustrator, Lisa Kroin, for lending her talents; to the amazing Dr. Judy Kuriansky for her support and guidance; to my editor, Alex Mummery, for her tireless efforts; and to my publicist, Tina Mosetis, for her incredibly hard work.

There are times when you take the hand

Life deals you,

And there are times when you deal the cards.

I say, who's playing

and

Let's deal.

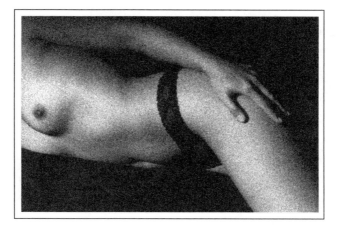

Between the Sheets with a Sexpert

A gentle sucking of the lips surrenders to a deeper kiss. A bra, then boxers, drop to the floor. You don't care that you're almost naked; you just want more. Body heat, this bed's on fire. You're burning hot with desire. Sexy thing, can't get enough. Harder. Faster. Yeah baby—rub!

Man, this is amazing! Girl, what a rush! You start to tense and tingle as your genitals are engorged with blood. Your body aches. Your nipples harden. Your crotch swells with anticipation. Feeling moist, getting hard. The air around you is supercharged, building for one of the sweetest sensations....

Bull's-eye—you feel—it's in! Your pelvis starts to grind as the penetration begins. Skin slapping in steady time. Thoughts, pure and profane, speed through your mind. Heart racing, blood pumping, you hear your breathing become gasping as every pulsation, every vibration gets stronger, hotter, more gripping, more intense...'til you think you'll lose control and your mind starts to go, and WAM!! You orgasm! And BAM!! You've hit heaven! And SHAZAM!! Now you're tripping. The room's full of colors; it won't stop spinning. And then come the tremors, and your entire being is exalted; the earth is still moving, and you think you just lost consciousness....

And you wake up with a smile. Shoot. It was just a dream. Your body is exhausted. You want to go back to sleep, back to that state of mind that's all about ecstasy. But you're feeling rather damp. Your sweaty pajamas are clinging to your skin, and you've got a wet spot again in your underpants. Worse yet, you realize that you're all alone; no one shares your bed. That class act was all solo, all just in your head. But who was the person in your dream? It doesn't really matter. You just hope that you'll have sex again sometime and wonder if maybe next time it'll be even better.

I take it I have your attention? Because that nocturnal dream was just a taste of all of the sexually charged material I want to cover with you in this book: sexual response, lust, hooking up, fantasy, orgasm. I have so much to tell you about sex, so much to share! We're getting into all of it!

We're going to delve into our sexual similarities, while looking at what makes us so deliciously unique and sexy: sexual desires, sexual stimuli, types of sex play, sexual scenarios, sexual expressions. In this book, we celebrate many of them; we eroticize many of them. In doing so, we also uphold a basic "sexploration" concern: taking care of our sexual health. For it is only when nurturing this part of our sexual selves that we can have—and completely lose ourselves in—the most incredible sex ever.

Yet, before we go any further, you may be wondering who am I to tell you about sex. What makes me such an authority on sex? I know I've asked the same of other self-proclaimed "sexperts": With so many people having sex in this world, what makes this person *the* expert? What can she tell me about sex that I don't already know?

I've been a sex educator since the sixth grade, when I shocked my wide-eyed, spellbound classmates with a formal, five-minute class presentation on the female reproductive system, menstruation, and sexual intercourse. With their eyes glued to the homemade clay model of a female's internal genitalia I used as my visual aid, I gave most of them what I am sure was their first lesson on sex. Thriving on their curiosity, intrigue, and attentiveness, I knew at that moment that I was destined to be a sex educator.

Twelve years after that class presentation, I graduated with a Master's degree in Human Sexuality Education from the University of Pennsylvania. Having had various courses dealing with the dysfunctions, behavioral foundations, biology, and concepts of sex, encompassing anything from different lifestyles, to various positions, to sexual assault, to STDs/HIV/AIDS, to pregnancy, to reproductive system cancers, to sexual orientation, I've been exposed to sexuality in a light even that good old sex bible *Cosmopolitan* has yet to see. This extensive educational background, flavored by my Scandinavian upbringing (I'm originally from Iceland), makes me an official "sexpert," seeking to disseminate knowledge and liberate our attitudes toward our sexual health, sex lives, and sexuality. I am currently working on my Ph.D. in International Community Health, with a sexual health focus. (If you'd like more information about me, check out my website: www.yvonnekfulbright.com)

Throughout my career, I have taught classes and given numerous workshops on sex topics like eroticizing safer sex, sexual behaviors, relationships, sexual assault, and HIV/AIDS, at both American and Canadian universities. In talking with fellow students, I have picked up on major themes in their questions and concerns. People want to know what other people are and aren't doing in the bedroom. They want numbers, statistics...solid, scientific sex facts! They want to know if something is too outrageous or kinky. They ask: What is normal? Is it okay to do this? What's the real scoop on *that*? What is *this* for? What does *that* do? What does *this* mean? Plus, young people want steamy sex tips on top of all of the practical information.

Attention: Calling All 20-Something-Year-Old Singles

This is the kind of book I wish that someone would've written for me—a hip, erotically charged, sexual survival guide of sorts that would've answered all of my questions regarding body parts, body image, contraception, STDs, HIV, orgasm, self-pleasuring, attraction, sexual positions, sexual enhancers, sexual health maintenance, and safer sex. So when, as a 23-year-old, I sat down to write this book, I envisioned it being for heterosexual 18- to 29-year-olds, though teenagers, singles over 30, and non-heterosexual individuals can benefit from its information as well. I thought about all of the things that you—my peers—might want to know, all of the things any sexually informed individual should know, and all of the things you *need* to know to have a healthy, better, safer sex life. With more young adults postponing marriage but maintaining active sex lives as singles, there's a lot we need to know to navigate some of the most socially thrilling, sexually liberating years of our lives.

Furthermore, in helping you become a savvy sexual being, we're going to make your safer-sex life incredibly erotic. In today's world, having unprotected sex is like playing a round of Russian roulette. You're taking a chance—one you may not walk away from unscathed. So no matter what you do when you're getting it on, you need to make sure that you're doing it responsibly and respectfully—if not for your life and your health, then for your partner's. Part of that involves using protection.

Keeping It Hot...

In practicing safer sex, many of my peers get concerned about how to keep things hot. So one of the main goals of this book is eroticizing safer sex—

using various physical and mental techniques, practices, and tricks that make protected sex absolutely out of this world. Much of the sex education we receive consists of "you can't do this" or "don't do that" messages, so we're left poorly equipped to protect our sexual health, let alone how to make sex safer and sensational. So consider this permission-giving book your license to safer sex, with major focus on the following:

*   How do I have "good" sex?

*   What can I do to absolutely blow my partner away?

*   What can I do to make sex more erotic and exciting?

*   How do I maintain a healthy sex life?

*   How does unsafe sex affect my health?

*   How do I protect myself?

*   How can I have *all* of that—do all of that?

I've divided the book's eighteen chapters into four sections, with illustrations and photos that enhance the text and visually explain sexual anatomy, body image, all types of pleasuring, contraceptives, sexual positions, and sex toys. In Part I, we're going to start with you and only you—the sexual you. I firmly believe that people need to focus on themselves, work on themselves, know, understand, accept, and love themselves before they can begin a fulfilling, healthy relationship with someone special. With a firm foundation about your sexual self, we're going to move into Part II, about sexual relationships and everything that being in one entails. We're going to cover what safer sex is all about before moving on to Part III. The third section is all about eroticizing safer sex. I'm going to give you some enticing, racy ways that you and your partner can make protected sex the best sex ever! In Part IV, I discuss two main factors that are threats to your sexual health: alcohol and drugs. Throughout the book, I combat a lot of myths about eroticizing sex and give tips on how to take care of yourself and your sexual health. Plus, I end each chapter with resources that offer you even more information.

Before I send you on your way, I want to bring special attention to the quotes you'll read throughout the book. The one constant I've found in being a sex educator over the years is that people need a sense of "normalcy" when it comes to sex, and I'm here to help you figure out what normal is for you. My social circle is here to give it to you. Not only do I give my take on a lot of sexual issues, but I have quotes from more than fifty 20-something-year-old people I know personally—friends, acquaintances, and coworkers—that tell you flat out what other people are doing and thinking between the sheets.

The reason I interviewed people I know personally is to demonstrate that if I know people who've tried this stuff, thought about this stuff, had an issue with this or that, desired this or that, then you probably know people like that too. Naturally, my quote contributors picked pseudonyms for themselves to protect their identity. This is some pretty juicy and sometimes hard-core stuff they're sharing!

I hope that you have a ball with this book. I'm psyched about all of the subject matter we're going to cover and all of the action we're going to see. I'd like to think that it will provide you with hours of entertainment. Sexual expression and affection are such a huge part of who we are, and we need to take care of our sexual selves, our sexual health. I'm pleased that in reading this book, you're seeking to do that. The following eighteen chapters are what it's all about.

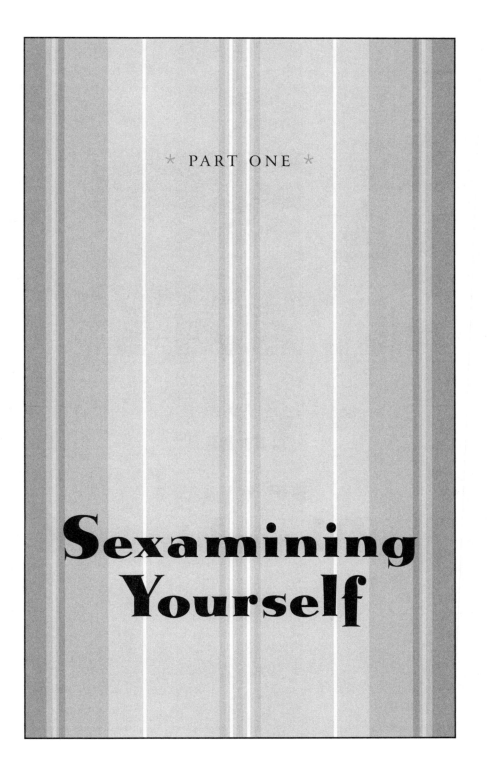

* PART ONE *

Sexamining Yourself

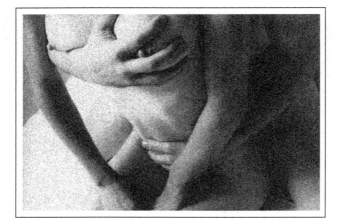

CHAPTER 1

Your Sexual Plumbing

Are you sexy? Can you feel sexier?

How can you become more comfortable with your body?

How does body image affect your sex life?

What makes up your sexual anatomy?

What happens to your body during sexual activity?

Before we get into anything that goes on when you're pulsating with pelvic passion, we have to begin with the sexiest thing you have going on—you! I hope you agree with me: *You* are the sexiest thing imaginable! You know that you're all that and then some. You've been feeling like one mega sex symbol lately. Watch out, world, this is one act you don't want to miss!

Okay, maybe that's a bit of an exaggeration. Naturally, we don't always feel so "modelesque" in our youthful, 20-something-year-old bodies. It's just that in my world you will see your body as beautiful, sexy, and head-turning attractive, whether it's because of the sparkle in your eye, the color of your sun-kissed hair, or your bright, winning smile. We've all got something about ourselves that's sexy, something to be proud of, and in this chapter we're going to get naked and show off our bodies. We're going to give new meaning to the term "self-examination." Part I of this book is devoted solely to you—how wonderful, beautiful, and sexual you are. We need to focus on you before we can worry about how you can share yourself with someone else. So let's take a better look at just how sexy you are!

The Battle of Body Image

In this day and age, it is by no means easy to have a positive body image, to see ourselves as beautiful. We're constantly battling damaging social conditioning and negative messages about what exactly makes a body beautiful. Most of us have it ingrained in us that we need a better body—a perfect body—in order to be attractive. We're constantly feeling that pressure, with the media and Hollywood mercilessly bombarding us with images of built beasts and starving vamps, all promoted as society's gorgeous, sexy elite.

In trying to feel good about our bodies, each and every one of us combats the media's prevailing idea of what is sexy and attractive, because most of us don't have what is hailed as the "perfect" physique—and never will. That's the bad news. The good news is that most of us are in the same boat on this one, so we're in this together—we're "not-so-perfect" together. Though it's hard, we have to get over comparing ourselves to societal standards, standards that are extremely unrealistic and often terribly unhealthy. It's got to stop. For the duration of this book, it will stop. We need to take charge and set our own standards of what is attractive. We do this by first challenging our negative thinking, and then by focusing on the beauty of the self.

BODY-IMAGE ISSUES

No matter how good we look, body-image issues are almost inescapable. Everybody has some body part about which they're unsure or insecure, or just not crazy about. That's a given; we're human. Like Kim, a 22-year-old graduate student, a young lady who has everything going for her but who still feels self-conscious about her chest at times:

> I wear a 34C and I'm 5'1" and about 120 pounds. My breasts seem to be bigger than those of the average girl my size, or so I've been told by guys. But this bothers me. I never felt my breasts were big, so to speak, until I started getting the jokes from my friends. I'm really insecure about it and I try not to wear things that emphasize them.

Johann is a 21-year-old business major. While he's a regular male Mary Poppins, practically perfect in every single way, he brings up one of the biggest male insecurities of all—penis size:

> I don't have anything to compare my penis size to. I don't have a problem with it, but then you see *Boogie Nights* and start to wonder.... Porn stars are hung like horses. I just wonder if I should have insecurities. I read *Maxim* and they tell you size doesn't matter. I don't know if they're trying to make you feel good. I hear women prefer girth to length. I don't know what the ideal size is.

Even if we don't have an issue with a body part, we wonder if we should. Body-image issues and insecurities suck. Furthermore, it's enough to deal with them on your own, but when you decide to fool around and get naked with somebody, these issues can really put a damper on things, making you self-conscious of your body and lovemaking. When you're exposing your every physical feature to someone, it's hard to escape the negativity and submerge yourself in your sexuality.

I take comfort in reminding myself that 89 percent of women and 72 percent of men are unhappy with at least one aspect of their appearance. Likewise, only 3 percent of men and women consider themselves a knockout. So quit being hard on yourself! If you take the time to really look at your body and all of its beauty, you'll soon see that you truly are a work of art.

BODY-IMAGE BASICS

Tuning into your sexuality and your sexual potential starts with body image and positive self-appraisal. Body comfort helps you to loosen up during sex and can lead to greater intimacy between yourself and your partner. Negative thoughts about being nude are the last things you should be worrying about during sex play. You have much more important things to focus on!

Learning to love your body—and love yourself—is key to a better sex life and a more sexual you. You have to be able to love yourself before you can love someone else. This will help you to be freer and less inhibited in bed, and that sets the stage for all of the rocket-launching sex play we're going to cover in this book.

Having a positive attitude and feelings about your physique includes getting in touch with your body, learning to appreciate it, and concentrating on your good parts. In dealing with your body image, you need to become more comfortable with your body, with nudity, and with being nude. You need to change your negative thinking and boost your self-esteem. These are the first and best things you can do for yourself and your sex life. So here are some body-image exercises for you...

BODY-IMAGE EXERCISES

1. Try walking around your bedroom nude. Choose a time when you can be alone and undisturbed—in your element. Relax! Soak

in how good it feels to be unclothed and unrestricted. You are in your most natural state, the way you were born. You're careless and free! Stretch. Breathe deeply. Spread yourself out on your bed and relax. Absorb the sensation of the sheets against your bare skin. Enjoy. How often do you have the chance to be totally naked? Nudity is a luxury not enjoyed enough by most people!

2. Eventually, work your way over to a full-length mirror and stand nude in front of it. Think about what you dislike about your body and why those areas bother you, for example, "I wish that I had a flat stomach."

3. Now combat those negative thoughts by thinking about *all* of the things you like about your body and why you like them. Tell yourself—out loud—what you love about your body, for example, "I've got nice shoulders" or "I love my butt—I had it going on long before J-Lo made it vogue!" Remember, you are the latest craze!

Frolicking nude around your room is just the beginning of a better body image. To feel good about yourself and your physique, take time out for yourself. As silly as it sounds, whether you're a male or female, make a date with yourself. You're always being nice to other people, lavishing gifts and good things on them. For once, pamper yourself, be good to your body. This kind of date with yourself can be anything solo you fancy that lets you get in touch with your body. This could be an invigorating yoga or tae kwon do session. You're slowly moving your muscles, getting in touch with your inner being, indulging in how good it feels to be you. Or your idea of an ideal date could be going on a nice, long run, thriving on the feeling of your muscles at work and the freedom a good pace can create.

You could also try treating yourself to a bubble bath, filled with your favorite scented oil. Allow yourself to totally relax and enjoy the warm steam rising off the water. Take the opportunity to explore your body; investigate every part. More than anything, relax and just luxuriate in your body's intended, unclothed form. Then, following the bath, rub lotion all over your body. Your skin craves moisture and it feels good to royally treat every inch of it with a nice, rich lotion. Plus, using a moisturizer helps to heal some of those rough, dry patches your fingertips might discover as they dance over your body. Not only is silky, baby smooth skin something you deserve, but it can be a turn-on for anybody who touches your body, yourself included. Next time you're with a partner, you'll feel so soft your lover won't be able to take his or her hands off your body. You'll feel better, too, as your partner's hands wander, knowing that you've got one sexy body.

When you're with your partner, convince yourself that your lover is thrilled with you and loves your body. After all, your partner must be attracted to you and dig your body or else your lover wouldn't be involved with you. Since you are his empress or her demigod, don't draw attention to what you dislike about your body—your partner may not have even noticed your "flaw." Keep your "imperfections" to yourself!

Insecurities are unattractive; confidence is what's sexy. Acting confident about yourself and your body will help you to feel sexier, to love your body, and to be proud of it. If you feel sexy, you will be sexy.

Now that you've gotten a body-image pep talk, we should take the next step toward better body image: getting to know yourself (and the opposite sex) inside and out. Pay close attention, since knowing these parts will help you later in the book.

Female Sexual Anatomy

EXTERNAL GENITALIA

The Vulva

The **vulva** (pudendum) is a collective term for the female external genitals: the clitoris, mons pubis, labia minora, labia majora, the urethral opening, and the vaginal opening (see the illustration on page 14). It is an erotic, sensitive area that protects the vagina and urethral opening.

The Clitoris

Since 50 to 75 percent of women need direct clitoral stimulation in order to reach orgasm during intercourse, the clitoris is by far the one part of the female anatomy you should know. The **clitoris** is a small, highly sensitive

External Female Genitalia

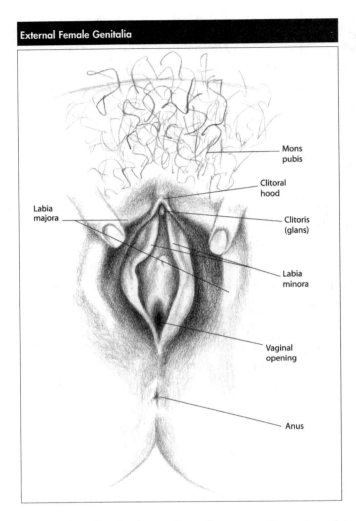

Mons pubis

Clitoral hood

Labia majora

Clitoris (glans)

Labia minora

Vaginal opening

Anus

sexual organ, filled with a high number of nerve endings, found *in front of* the vaginal entrance and urethra (some people mistake the urethra for the clitoris). It is protected by a sheath of tissue—the **clitoral hood**—that passes around the clitoris and is an extension of the inner lips that run alongside the vaginal opening.

> The clitoris has absolutely no known purpose other than to provide the female with pleasure! It's anywhere from three-quarters of an inch to 1¼ inches long. When sexually excited or stimulated, the clitoris fills with blood and becomes hard—"erect"—and doubles in size.

The clitoris has two parts: the shaft, which disappears into the body beneath the clitoral hood, and the glans, the visible, external tip that protrudes like a small lump. The glans is the part of the woman's genitals that is most sensitive to touch.

The Mons Pubis

The **mons pubis** is that fatty pad of tissue and skin under a woman's pubic hair, over her pubic bone. It protects the pubic bones from damage during vigorous sexual thrusting and, in some women, is sensitive to sexual stimulation.

The Labia Majora/Labia Minora

The outer lips and inner lips together make up the woman's labia. The **labia majora** (outer lips) are rounded pads of fibrous, fatty tissue, covered with pubic hair, lying on either side of the vaginal entrance. They contain glands that produce the odorous sweat that is a natural, sexual chemical attractant.

The **labia minora** (inner lips) are thin, hairless folds of skin lying on either side of the vaginal entrance. They have glands that produce sebum, which lubricates the skin and, when combined with the secretions from the vagina and sweat glands, forms a waterproof protective covering.

The labia minora are an erogenous body part to pay attention to since they're highly sensitive to touch. Labia vary from woman to woman in size, color, and shape.

The Urethral Opening

The **urethral opening** is an acorn-shaped protrusion found between the clitoris and vaginal opening. It's filled with nerve endings, and stimulation of it can evoke feelings ranging from highly arousing to unpleasant, or can feel like nothing at all.

Vaginal Opening

The **vaginal opening**, which leads to the woman's vagina, is the opening through which a baby passes during birth and through which menstrual blood passes during her period. During sexual intercourse, the penis is inserted into the vagina via the vaginal opening.

Bartholin's Glands

Bartholin's glands are small glands on either side of the vaginal opening. They secrete a small amount of fluid during sexual stimulation.

Skene's Glands

Skene's glands are the female's urethral glands. They secrete female ejaculatory fluid in women who ejaculate. (For more information on female ejaculation, see Chapter 12.)

Breasts

The **breasts** are the secondary sex organs found on a woman's chest. Each breast is composed of fatty and fibrous tissue that surrounds fifteen to twenty clusters of mammary glands, each of which has a separate opening to the **nipple** and is capable of producing milk. The nipple of the breast is surrounded by the round, darkened area called the **areola**, which consists of smooth muscle fibers that cause the nipple to become erect. An areola may be any shade of brown, black, or pink and any shape—protruding, flat, or inverted.

A woman's breasts are not always the same size. One is usually slightly larger.

INTERNAL GENITALIA

The Vagina

The **vagina** is a highly muscular, tube-shaped organ in the female into which the penis is inserted during sex between a woman and a man, and through which a baby passes during birth. It is a passageway that connects the vaginal opening and the cervix. It is three to four inches long, with most of its nerves in its lower third.

The vaginal walls rest against each other when in an unaroused state, but upon arousal, they expand outward and become lubricated.

The Hymen

The hymen is a thin tissue membrane that covers the opening of the vagina. It usually stretches across some, but not all, of the vaginal opening and is perforated (this allows menstrual blood to go through). It has no known function.

Female internal anatomy

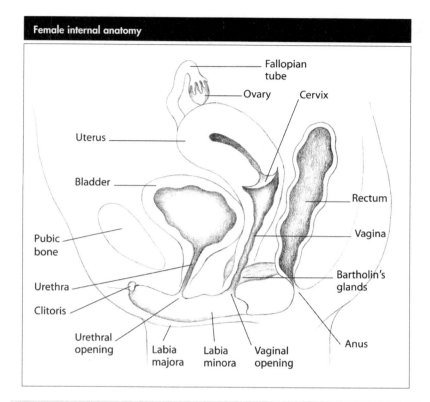

Often, societies mistake the presence of an intact hymen as proof of a female's virginity. Having a hymen does not necessarily mean that the woman is a virgin and not having a hymen does not mean that the woman is not a virgin. The presence or absence of an intact hymen is not an accurate indication of a female's sexual past. Her hymen can be broken, torn, or stretched at early ages by various exercises or by inserting fingers or objects into her vagina, e.g., tampons. Some women are even born with only a partial hymen or none at all. In addition, sexual intercourse doesn't always tear the hymen and may simply stretch it.

The Cervix

The **cervix** is the opening to the uterus. It consists of a **cervical os**, the very small cervical opening that will not allow a penis, sex toy, tampon, or finger to enter the uterus, yet will stretch enough for the insertion of medical instruments and opens during ovulation, menstruation, and labor.

For most women, the cervix is more responsive to pressure than to touch since it has few nerve endings. Some women find pressure of the penis on the cervix during sex lovely, while others may find it quite painful, especially if some hard thrusting is going on. Usually, a woman will be aware of her cervix during deep penile thrusting.

The Uterus

About the size of a fist, the **uterus** is the hollow, muscular organ located in the abdomen. It contains and nourishes the developing embryo and fetus during pregnancy. It consists of the **body** (upper portion) and the **cervix** and is composed of three layers. The endometrium is the inner layer, or uterine lining, that thickens with blood and then sloughs off when a woman has her menstrual period.

The Fallopian Tubes

The **fallopian tubes** extend from the uterus to the ovaries. One tube extends about four inches from each side of the uterus, with ends, called **fimbrae**, that look like flower petals. The tubes are lined with cilia that help to move the egg toward the uterus after it has been released from the ovary, caught by the fimbrae, and begun its venture down the fallopian tube.

The Ovaries

About the size of almonds, the two **ovaries** are organs that release eggs at ovulation and the sex hormones estrogen and progesterone. They are the female's primary sex organs. The ovaries are found at the ends of the fallopian tubes, on either side of the uterus. They store the 400,000 eggs a female possesses at birth. Only about 400 of these eggs are released during a woman's lifetime.

The Urethra and Urethral Sponge

The **urethra** is a slender tube that acts as a passageway for urine making its way out of the body. It is surrounded by spongy, erectile tissue called the **"urethral sponge"** or **"G-spot"** (for a detailed discussion on the G-spot and where to find it, see Chapter 12), which contains the paraurethral glands and ducts. The size of the tissue, and the paraurethral glands it contains, varies from woman to woman.

Male Sexual Anatomy

EXTERNAL GENITALIA

The Penis

The **penis** is the male reproductive and sex organ. Its reproductive purpose is to pass sperm into the vagina. It also passes urine out of the body. The penis is composed of several sections. The **glans** is the smooth, extremely sensitive tip that contains numerous nerve endings. The **root** is the part of the penis that attaches to the body. The **body**, or **shaft**, runs between the two. The penis is covered with muscles (yet the penis itself is not a muscle) and is filled with a rich network of blood vessels and blood spaces that have the potential to fill with blood and expand during erection.

The **corona** is a raised ridge separating the glans from the body of the penis and is the most sexually excitable region of the penis. The **frenulum** is a tiny band of skin near the indentation on the underside of the penis,

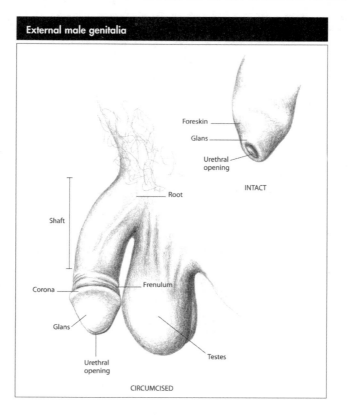

External male genitalia

Foreskin
Glans
Urethral opening
INTACT

Root
Shaft
Corona
Frenulum
Glans
Urethral opening
Testes
CIRCUMCISED

where the glans meets the shaft. It is an extremely sensitive part of the penis and reacts quickly to arousal. On men who are uncircumcised, you'll find a **foreskin**—the layer of skin covering the glans, which retracts when the male is aroused and erect.

> Starting from where the penis shaft protrudes from the groin, and running along the undersurface of the penis, the average flaccid (non-erect) penis is two to four inches in length. An erect penis length is $4^5/_8$ to $6^1/_4$ inches, with the average girth being about $4^3/_4$ inches. (This is what most women estimate it to be.) Anywhere within an inch of that range is considered mainstream, with 12 percent of the population exceeding that range and 12 percent falling under it. Smaller flaccid penises increase more in size during erection than do larger flaccid penises.

The Scrotum

The **scrotum** is a pouch of dark, thin skin, containing numerous sebaceous glands and covered in hair, that holds and protects the **testes**, a pair of glands that manufacture sperm and testosterone. Found below the root of the penis, the scrotum also regulates the temperature of the testes, since sperm must be produced at five degrees lower than body temperature. The scrotum regulates temperature by sweating and by contracting muscles that bring the testes closer to the body (to increase temperature) or by relaxing muscles to lower the testes away from the body (to reduce temperature).

INTERNAL GENITALIA

The Testes

The **testes** are a pair of oval glands—**gonads**—in the scrotum, which manufacture sperm and sex hormones, primarily testosterone. Also known as the **testicles**, each of these male reproductive glands is $1^1/_2$ inches in size and contains hundreds of tiny coiled tubes—**seminiferous tubules**—that produce sperm. About 300,000 sperm are produced in each ejaculation.

> Usually the left testicle hangs lower than the right, to avoid the two whacking into each other, and one may even be slightly larger than the other in some men.

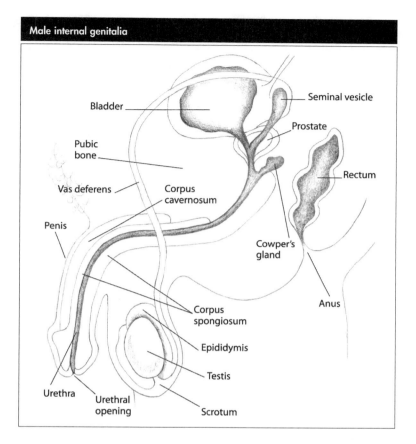

Male internal genitalia

Bladder

Seminal vesicle

Prostate

Pubic bone

Rectum

Vas deferens

Corpus cavernosum

Penis

Cowper's gland

Anus

Corpus spongiosum

Epididymis

Testis

Urethra

Urethral opening

Scrotum

The Prostate Gland

The size of a chestnut, the **prostate** is a gland found under the bladder, behind the pubic bone, that secretes some of the milky, alkaline fluid in semen. This fluid helps with sperm movement and protects sperm from the acidity of the woman's vagina and the man's urethra during sex. The prostate is composed of both glandular and muscle tissue and surrounds the prostate urethra.

The Seminal Vesicles

Found at the base of the bladder, the **seminal vesicles** are two small sacs that produce and secrete about 60 percent of the thick, rich-in-sugar (specifically fructose, the sugar commonly found in fruit) ejaculate fluid—**semen**.

The Epididymis

The **epididymis** is a tightly coiled, thin tube that lies alongside and on top of each of the testicles. Sperm move through these two tubes on their way out into the penis, and as they do so, the epididymides secrete a small amount of fluid that will help the sperm cells finish maturing. Sperm can be stored in the epididymides for up to six weeks to grow and mature.

The Vas Deferens

The **vas deferens** are tubes that transport sperm to the seminal vesicles and prostate gland from the epididymides.

The Bulbourethral Glands

Men have two pea-sized glands on either side of their urethra, within the penis, called **bulbourethral glands**, or **Cowper's glands**. When sexually aroused, these glands secrete a clear, alkaline fluid into the urethra that appears at the tip of the penis before a male ejaculates—"**pre-cum**" or "**pre-ejaculatory fluid.**"

In Both Sexes

THE PERINEUM

The **perineum** is the soft tissue between the vaginal opening or testes and the anus. This area is composed of spongy, erectile tissue and is where many pelvic-floor muscles crisscross each other. Since it's connected to the pudendal nerve, it is a highly erogenous area of the body.

Isn't it marvelous how our bodies are so well put together?! Everything has a purpose. If you haven't already, take the time to examine your genitalia with a handheld mirror. Get up close and personal with yourself. Check this stuff out! Your genitalia is really quite like nothing else. You can even have a good time checking yourself out with a partner, showing off your every feature. Your partner will think it's a crime that you look so good and will be turned on enough to take you on the ride of your life—right through the sexual response cycle.

Your Sexual Response Cycle

Before we get into your red-hot, mattress-melting, sexual adventures, it's a good idea to become familiar with what fuels your fire, what makes it all possible—your **sexual response cycle**. Knowing this cycle can help you to better understand your body's physiological reactions to sexual arousal and make you more comfortable with these natural bodily responses. It's the kind of knowledge that can help you love your "sexca-pades" that much more.

One great thing about the sexual response cycle that makes it all the more worthwhile to become familiar with is that it can be just as powerful, just as amazing, when practicing safer sex—a term you're going to hear a lot throughout this book—as when not. **Safer sex** is vaginal, anal, or oral sex involving practices that reduce the risk of contracting HIV and STDs and the chance of getting pregnant. Such practices reduce the amount of body fluids (semen, vaginal fluids, breast milk, and blood) that are passed from partner to partner. Such sex is called *safer* sex because, although it does greatly reduce the risk of disease transmission, it doesn't totally elim-inate the risk.

Safer sex is the only effective way, other than **abstinence** (defined here as refraining from all sexual activity that involves the exchange of body fluids) to protect yourself—and your partner—from the negative conse-quences of sex. Many people have a bad attitude about safer sex. They complain that it reduces sensation, interferes with intimacy, and requires too much planning and effort. This book challenges people with this mentality to think otherwise. Knowing the ins and outs of your body and the nitty-gritty details of your sexual response cycle are just a couple of ways you can train your body and mind to embrace safer sex without sacri-ficing any of the sensations that make you moan.

The sexual response cycle is basically a template of what generally happens to men and women when they're engaging in sexual activity. I must point out, however, that all of the physiological responses outlined here do not necessarily occur in every aroused individual. For example, not every woman's nipples become erect when she's being stimulated—and there's nothing wrong with that.

So don't think that you're abnormal if your body's reactions don't fit this cycle to a T. There is, though, a general pattern of physiological and psychological functions, known as your sexual response cycle, that holds up for every human being, and is worth knowing about and quite arousing in itself!

There are four stages your body goes through during the sexual response cycle: excitement, plateau, orgasm, and resolution. During the first three of these four stages, the following two basic physiological processes occur:

* **vasocongestion**—the accumulation of blood in the blood vessels of a region of the body, especially the genitals and breasts
* **myotonia**—muscle contraction

The four stages, based on these two reactions to sexual stimuli, are what make the human body so incredible, so sexual, and so capable of producing its own supercharged, natural experience of flying 14,000 feet up and getting ready for your first sky dive.

Sex for Physical Benefits

Whether they orgasm or not, sex helps men and women to relax and promotes a healthy heart. It can shield the body from illness and the mind from depression or aggression. Sex once a week or more promotes a regular menstrual cycle in women whose cycles are irregular, improves women's fertility, and promotes healthier bones.

William Masters and Virginia Johnson were the first sexologists to study the sexual response cycle in the 1960s and it has been further researched by others ever since. Some professionals present five stages to the sexual response cycle, while others stick with the original four given by Masters and Johnson. The difference in the number of cycle stages has to do with desire.

Desire is the factor that some people think is its own separate stage and that others choose to consider part of the excitement phase of the cycle. Regardless of where it fits in, in order for the sexual response cycle to begin, you need desire. You need to tap into your innate psychological drive, that part of you that's full of appetite, instinct, and lust. This is not always an easy thing to do. Sometimes your desire is affected by your self-confidence, health, tension, fatigue, hormone levels, work, etc. Ultimately, whenever you get caught up in your sexual needs, desire becomes excitement. Your entire being is a state of energy!

EXCITEMENT

This first stage of the sexual response cycle, also known as the **arousal stage**, is the beginning of erotic arousal. Such arousal could be due to watching a porn film, to reading a romance novel, to feeling his hand on the inside of your upper thigh, to imagining your face between her heaving, perky breasts. At this stage the following things happen:

Men—Your penis fills with blood and becomes erect. The skin on your scrotum thickens as your scrotal sac tenses and pulls itself up closer to your body. Your spermatic cords shorten, pulling your testes closer to your body as well. Your breasts may swell and even enlarge, and your nipples may become erect.

Women—About ten to thirty seconds after arousal begins, your vagina begins to swell and lubricate. Your clitoris fills with blood and swells, becoming erect. Your inner lips also thicken, open up, deepen in color, and swell, doubling or tripling in size! The upper two-thirds of your vagina expands dramatically—a "ballooning" type of response takes place and your cervix and uterus pull up. Your nipples become erect and your breasts swell and enlarge somewhat, too.

Both Sexes—A *"sex flush"* takes place—your body blushes due to the increase in your pulse rate and blood pressure. Your heart rate works its way up to about 160 beats per minute. Your muscles tense and you're more sensitive to stimulation.

PLATEAU

This is the second stage of sexual response, just before orgasm, when you become increasingly aroused. Vasocongestion reaches its peak.

Men—Your penis becomes completely erect and your glans swells. Your testes are soooo engorged with blood that they may be up to 50 percent larger than they are in an unaroused state. Furthermore, they're now pulled up even higher and closer to your body. A few drops of fluid, pre-cum, appear at the tip of your penis.

Women—Your body prepares itself for orgasm with the formation of an **orgasmic platform**—the thickening of the walls of the outer third of your vagina. Your uterus becomes fully elevated. The size of your vaginal entrance becomes smaller and there may be a noticeable increase in your vagina's gripping of his penis or fingers. Your clitoris also draws itself up into the body and becomes almost numb with excitement.

Both Sexes—Your breathing, pulse rate, and blood pressure increase dramatically—they're almost *soaring!!*

Sex and Bonding

Sex promotes bonding in that hormones triggered by sex affect the brain and body. The downfall of this reaction is that you could fall in love with or become addicted to someone you don't even like or want in your life.

ORGASM

Orgasm is an intense sensation that occurs at the peak of sexual arousal and is followed by the release of sexual tensions. It consists of a series of rhythmic contractions of the pelvic muscles at 0.8-second intervals. Physiologically, orgasm is the shortest phase of the sexual response cycle, but psychologically, it can create the sense of momentary suspension in time, full of warm, electric, and/or tingly sensations that throb and race throughout the body.

Men—Your orgasm occurs in two stages. First, during the **preliminary stage (emission phase)**, the vas deferens, seminal vesicles, and prostate contract, forcing ejaculate into the bulb at the base of the urethra. This is when "**ejaculatory inevitability**" occurs—the sensation that ejaculation is just about to happen and can't be stopped. Smooth muscles all over your reproductive system contract, causing the seminal fluids to move into the widening urethra at the base of your penis.

Second, during the **expulsion phase**, the muscles at the base of your penis and your urethral bulb contract rhythmically, forcing your semen through the urethra and out of the opening at the tip of the penis. In order for this to occur, during ejaculation the neck of the urinary bladder is shut tightly to make sure that there is no mixing of urine and semen. After ejaculation, a small amount of semen is usually still in your urethra, to be expelled either when you urinate or if you gently "milk" the penis once your erection has gone down.

Women—Your pelvic and anal muscles contract rhythmically. The uterus contracts as well, with contractions moving in waves from the top of the uterus down to the cervix. Your sex flush reaches its greatest intensity. (Female orgasm will be covered in greater detail in Chapter 2.)

Both Sexes—There is a sharp increase in your pulse rate, blood pressure, and breathing rate during orgasm. All of the muscles throughout your body are contracting.

Sex and Touch

Physical touch enables the body to relax and feel protected and comfortable. For women, touch boosts oxytocin levels in the body. Oxytocin is a hormone that promotes care-taking behavior and feelings of affection.

RESOLUTION

This is the fourth and final stage of the sexual response cycle, during which your body returns to its unaroused state.

Men—The loss of your erection—**detumescence**—happens in two stages. The first stage occurs rapidly, but the penis remains somewhat enlarged as the blood leaves it. The second stage occurs more slowly, as more blood leaves the penis. Then, a **refractory period** settles in—a period following ejaculation during which you cannot be sexually aroused. During this time, you will be incapable of being aroused again, having an erection, or having an orgasm. You're all alone on this one. Women don't enter this state.

Women—The first change in your body is the reduction of the swelling of the breasts. About five to ten seconds after the end of orgasm, your clitoris returns to its normal position, though it takes longer for it to shrink to its normal size. Your orgasmic platform is relaxing. The ballooning of your vagina diminishes and your uterus shrinks. All of this takes about fifteen to thirty minutes total, but with the right kind of arousal, you can be hurled back into earlier stages of the cycle and experience the ride all over again, and quite rapidly at that!

Both Sexes—Your sex flush disappears rapidly. There is a gradual return of your unaroused blood pressure, pulse rate, and breathing rate levels.

Sex as Medicine

Sex in the context of a loving relationship, full of intimacy and closeness, boosts the chemicals in the body that protect you against disease. Sexual activity relieves pain in our joints and muscles due to chronic conditions, like arthritis and lower back pain, plus eases menstrual cramps for women.

Most people want to fall asleep within one hour after sex. Post-sex touching—**afterplay**—is strongly correlated with how satisfied both men and women feel about their relationships. Ironically, most members of both sexes are not completely satisfied with what goes on between the two of them after sex. This is mostly because we're ignorant as to what's really going on emotionally and physically after orgasm.

The ignorance is simply due to a lack of communication in the relationship. The fatigue is due to orgasm being a parasympathetic nervous response that causes a deep feeling of relaxation, especially for the male.

Why more so for the male? Women take longer to come down from sex than men. Besides the rapid loss of an erection, a man's heartbeat and breathing return to normal much sooner than a woman's since her body remains in a plateau state much longer after orgasm. So that's why a guy becomes sleepier sooner following sex, leaving his lovely lady feeling slightly disturbed and unloved as he rolls over to crash. Understanding that his fatigue is a normal physiological reaction could prevent a lot of unnecessary arguments, but certainly isn't an excuse for him not giving her at least a little bit of loving before drifting off to sleep.

Sex as Exercise

Every time you make love, you burn 100 to 150 calories—depending on how vigorous you are in bed! That's about the same as a brisk twenty-minute walk. Women, you can use up even more calories if you saddle up and ride on top during intercourse.

All in all, becoming more familiar with every inch of your body is going to make you more confident about your body, your health, and your sex life. Seeing yourself as attractive is going to make your sexual being absolutely dynamite! Knowing how your sexual response cycle works is going to help you feel more comfortable with your body's reactions to getting turned on, plus it will make you more confident in your safer-sex talents. With that, you're good to go for the rest of this book.

CHAPTER 2

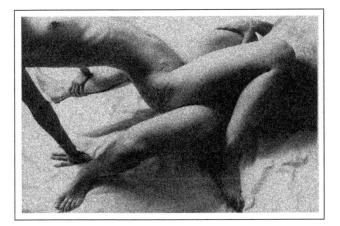

Orgasm!...
or
"I've Died and Gone to Heaven"

What is an orgasm? What does one feel like?

What are the different kinds of orgasm?

Why do we orgasm?

Why are some women multi-orgasmic?

Can men be multi-orgasmic?

Why do people fake orgasm?

What Is an Orgasm?

The best kind of orgasm is when you don't know whether to laugh or cry afterwards. An orgasm is the pinnacle of human emotion—it's ecstasy, release, connection, passion, all rolled into one. And besides, it feels damn good!" And that's only one person's way of describing orgasm. Orgasm is an out-of-body experience. It's ethereal. It's zing! Boom! Wow! Bam! Jeepers, Batman! You feel exalted.

Basically, an **orgasm** is a series of involuntary muscular contractions and a feeling of intense pleasure focused in the genitals that may spread throughout the body. It's your body's release of neuromuscular tension and of the blood that has rushed to your genitals during arousal. Orgasm's muscular contractions occur mostly in the pelvic region, including the rectal area, in both sexes. On average, an orgasm lasts three to ten seconds, with your genitals contracting up to fifteen times during that seemingly eternal time period.

There is no "right" or "wrong" way for somebody to have an orgasm. Sometimes you'll have incredible orgasms, sometimes they will be just OK, and sometimes they might not even happen. The experience of orgasm can be different every time and over time throughout your life. The sensations and orgasm you might have felt as a youth are going to be different from the ones you now revel in as a 20-something-year-old, and these will continue to evolve as you age and have different life experiences.

For some people, orgasm is attained as a result of genital stimulation, while for others it may occur just through nipple stimulation, massages, or even fantasy. Mood, level of energy, fatigue, level of partner trust, amount and type of foreplay and stimulation, and life events all have effects on the sensation of orgasm and our ability to "achieve" it. Furthermore, everyone has the potential to orgasm, but not everyone does.

Men and Orgasm

In men, there are two kinds of orgasm: a **penis-induced orgasm** and a **prostate-triggered orgasm**. For most men, orgasm is almost always achieved entirely through penis stimulation (see Chapter 12 for more information on the prostate-triggered orgasm). The onset of orgasm originates in a man's prostate, moving into his penis and testicles, and may then spread to become an entire body experience. It is almost, but not always, accompanied by the ejaculation of semen, since orgasm and ejaculation are two separate functions. An orgasm is simply the involuntary contraction of the pelvic muscles and that temporary state of ecstasy, while ejaculation is the emission of semen out of the penis.

During an orgasm, a man's penis is in a throbbing, erect state that produces about four to five warm, rhythmic contractions. These awesome sensations are experienced before the semen is forced up the urethra and ejaculated. When a man ejaculates, he experiences the warmth of the semen spurting or shooting out of his urethra.

Some men may experience their orgasm quietly, but contort their faces, while others may moan, groan, and thrash around loudly. For most, the intensity of the experience falls between these two extremes. A man's thrusting may become very intense and his breathing may become very hard, or his body may shudder with contractions as he holds his breath. Even after the main, most powerful contraction of orgasm is attained, the man may have sensations of orgasm for a long time afterward.

Women and Orgasm

The duration and intensity of an orgasm differs from woman to woman and from time to time. Some women experience an intense peak of pleasure that quickly fades, while others experience a longer-lasting, gradually spreading warmth. Others have a peak orgasm and then gradually subside into a series of smaller orgasms. Mason, a 23-year-old who loves to sport high heels, describes her orgasms:

> I never know what to expect as far as my orgasms go. My orgasmic experience can be as light as a few pleasurable, pelvic pulses, to one mind-blowing, powerful orgasm, to entire body-rocking multiple orgasms that grip and possess my entire being. A lot of it has to do with the kind of stimulation that's going on, the amount of privacy during sexual activity, sounds being made, my lover's skills, the use of fantasy....
> No matter what happens, the orgasm is never a disappointment!

During orgasm, a woman's body may arch, her muscles may tense, and her face may contort. She might scream, bite her lips, or cry out in pleasure, or she may just be quiet. Some women, after having had an orgasm, may even drift into a mild form of unconsciousness known as "little death."

TYPES OF FEMALE ORGASM

Research shows that women can attain at least three types of orgasm: clitoral, vaginal, and a combination of the two. Most women attain orgasm by having their clitoris stimulated—a **clitoral orgasm**. Some women may reach an intense, deep orgasm—a **vaginal orgasm**—that involves their uterus and reproductive system muscles, especially if only their G-spot is stimulated. A third type of woman orgasms from having their clitoris and vagina stimulated at the same time. This combination type of orgasm results in the most powerful orgasm of the three. Some women report that having a finger inserted into the rectum near the time of orgasm intensifies the sensation during any of these orgasms as well.

Fifty to seventy-five percent of orgasmic women do not experience an orgasm if penile thrusting is the only form of stimulation.

WHY DOES A WOMAN ORGASM?

The biological purpose of a male's orgasm is pretty obvious—it's a means of projecting sperm into the vagina so that fertilization can take place. Yet for decades, researchers have wondered why women orgasm. The reason is not as obvious nor as functional as for the male. So what is the purpose of a female orgasm?

Researchers have only been able to speculate about this. One popular notion is that female orgasm is a mechanism that improves the chances of the male's sperm reaching the female's egg. If a woman climaxes before or up to forty-five minutes after her male lover ejaculates, or if her orgasm happens before his by more than a minute, she retains significantly more sperm than she does after nonorgasmic sex. Other research findings have been just as intriguing. A woman's ability to orgasm depends *not* on her partner's skills, but on her subconscious evaluation of his genetic potential. Women whose partners have the most symmetrical physical features enjoy a significantly higher frequency of orgasm during sexual intercourse (but not during foreplay or other sexual activities) than do those with less symmetrical partners. Orgasm, in many respects, is sort of a smart trick of nature to ensure survival of the fittest, the genetically healthiest humans.

WHAT'S LOVE GOT TO DO WITH IT?

It may come as a surprise that a woman's orgasm has *little* to do with love or experience. Women aren't any more built for monogamy than men are—they're programmed to keep their options open. Neither the amount of a woman's romantic attachment for her partner, nor the partner's sexual experience, increase the frequency of her orgasm. As nice as it sounds, being in love with her well-experienced stallion *is not* going to make her orgasm any more intensely than hard-core sex with a stranger would.

While research findings like these are fun and do offer some insight as to why women orgasm, I wouldn't plan my sex life or my desire to have an orgasm around them. A woman's ability to orgasm involves a lot more than biological instinct. Female orgasm is a very individual thing. For Demi, a 22-year-old youth rights advocate, it's about sex being a heart-to-heart experience: "When you have an orgasm with someone you love, it's as though you become one, pulsing against each other. The feeling is hard to describe, but it's almost like you're in another state of mind and very free to express your innermost physical feelings with that person."

A woman's orgasm is dependent on a woman's ability to surrender to sensations, to her body, and to her own sexuality. It's about trusting her partner and being able to let go with him, in front of him. Plus, it's about the erogenous zones we have all over our bodies, finding out where they are, and knowing what sensations turn us on. For example, one woman I know can orgasm simply by having the palms of her hands stroked!

Simultaneous Orgasm

Fireworks. Cosmic collisions. Two tight bodies, feeling every part of an explosive orgasm in perfect rhythm. Every now and then, a couple will actually have a simultaneous orgasm—and quite accidentally at that. **Simultaneous orgasm** occurs when a man's thrusting slows down a bit and a woman's sexual response cycle speeds up a tad (since males usually orgasm first) so that they meet in the middle and orgasm at the same time. Since simultaneous orgasm is an exception in lovemaking, it can be rather exhausting for the goal-oriented couple who works toward it every time they have sex.

Simultaneous orgasm can be a really amazing experience since it happens only on occasion, but it is not something that should be deemed the pinnacle of making love. Half the fun of having sex is being able to watch your partner have an orgasm, and that cannot be done too well if you're caught up in your own!

Spontaneous Orgasm

A few lucky women (less than 10 percent), and even fewer men, are able to experience **spontaneous orgasm** (**extragenital orgasm**), which occurs with *no* genital contact. Instead, people who have this type of orgasm can sometimes excite themselves with erotic thoughts and fantasies to the point that any form of physical stimulation, like touching their earlobes, thigh, or neck, sends them over the edge. Topanga, a 25-year-old, sensual French sales rep, is one of the fortunate when it comes to spontaneous orgasm: "I can orgasm from just kissing a guy. All I have to do is cross my legs and just squeeze while he's kissing me. I'm that turned on!"

Sometimes, spontaneous orgasm is reached solely through concentration and mind control. Women who do orgasm spontaneously report that it occurs most often while doing a particular form of exercise, like aerobics or sit-ups, or after they've already had an orgasm produced by genital touching.

> Our brain is our biggest sex organ. Even individuals whose genitals have been removed for one reason or another can have orgasms. Never underestimate the power of your mind!

Nocturnal Orgasm

Another type of orgasm is the one that happens when you least expect it, when you can least control it, when you're dead asleep. Better known as "**wet dreams**," these **nocturnal orgasms** are all about your mind. Your brain gets your body so worked up that you go through the sexual response cycle while you're sleeping, often to the point of orgasm. More often than not, the only evidence of orgasm for a male is the ejaculation of semen, and for a female, it's a wet spot in her underwear, if that. The whole phenomenon is smashing, proving that your brain is your biggest sex organ.

WHAT CAUSES NOCTURNAL ORGASM?

Nocturnal orgasms can be the result of any stimulus your brain conjures up during sleep. Your mind doesn't hold back whatsoever, reeling out sensual situations, sultry scenery, and sex as you've never known it before—and may never know it again. Byron, a 24-year-old frustrated businessman, recalls what turns him on at night: "I've had wet dreams about specific women I know, women I'm dating. They're awesome! In my mind, it's like the feeling that you're in a dream and falling off a cliff. I never die in those kinds of dreams. In my wet dreams, I'm never done having sex. I always wake up right when I orgasm. It's surreal, confusing, and then over...."

Sometimes, your dreams and nocturnal orgasm can really surprise you, as Ashley, a 23-year-old health educator, learned:

> One night, I woke up in the middle of an incredible orgasm. My upper body was flying up into a sitting position as I was orgasming in my sleep. Right away, I orgasmed a couple of more times—really hard. As soon as my head hit my pillow again, I was out. The only reason I know it happened is because I vaguely remembered it the next morning, even wondering if it had really happened, since I was so surprised.

Multiple Orgasms

WHY DO WOMEN HAVE MULTIPLE "O'S"?

Multiple orgasms are a series of orgasms that occur within a short period of time. If a woman is stimulated again and again, she can immediately be aroused and move back into the excitement or plateau phase of her sexual response cycle and have another orgasm. So instead of moving into the "resolution," or final stage of orgasm, a woman can move back into the plateau phase after one orgasm and, with further stimulation, can experience a third orgasm, a tenth orgasm, a fifteenth orgasm....

Some women say that multiple orgasms occur through sexual intercourse, while others say that they occur more frequently via clitoral stimulation during masturbation, due to the ease of sexual stimulation, the lack of distraction due to partner concerns, greater use of sexual fantasy, and heightened breast and vaginal awareness. All women have the capability to experience multiple orgasms, but less than 50 percent actually have them.

While multiple orgasms are a bonus to any sexual rendezvous, there are women who do not experience multiple orgasms and who are perfectly satisfied with their sex lives. Lise, a 24-year-old medical student, exclaims: "I don't like the stereotype of women and multiple orgasms. After I have one orgasm, I'm pretty much done. I don't like the pressure on women that it's normal and easy to have an orgasm. I don't know if that's always the case for every woman."

WHAT MAKES SOME WOMEN MORE MULTI-ORGASMIC THAN OTHERS?

There are some notable differences between women who are multi-orgasmic and those who are not. Multi-orgasmic women

* tend to be more sexually adventurous and have greater sexual desire.

* are more likely to use clitoral stimulation via thigh pressure and to use vaginal stimulation with finger penetration during masturbation.

❈ have more frequently explored a variety of other techniques for experiencing orgasm, such as using a vibrator, sexual fantasies, or erotic materials, to become sexually excited.

❈ have also performed more sexual behaviors with a partner (like oral sex), have stimulated herself or had her partner stimulate her clitoris during sexual intercourse, and have had finger and oral stimulation of her nipples.

❈ have partners with whom they're able to communicate their needs.

❈ often experience their first orgasm before their male partner reaches orgasm!

I must point out the important role men can sometimes play in making a woman experience multiple orgasms. Let's take Jack and Jill, for example. If Jack uses deep and rapid thrusting when they make love, Jill is more likely to be multi-orgasmic. By masturbating Jill or by using a vibrator on her, Jack further increases Jill's chances of having more than one orgasm. Yet one of the biggest ways Jack can help Jill have multiple orgasms during sex is by exercising his own careful control in avoiding ejaculation. By delaying it, Jack helps Jill to "catch up" to his level of arousal; being stimulated for a prolonged period of time, while having sex, will help her have multiple orgasms.

So You've Never Had an Orgasm?

Anorgasmia is the inability to have an orgasm, whether the woman has never had an orgasm or has lost her ability to have one. A female may not be able to orgasm due to a variety of biological and cultural factors, including the following:

❈ fatigue

❈ tightness of muscles

❈ a partner's inability to satisfy her sexually

❈ having given into pressure to have sex before she's ready

❈ negative messages about sex while growing up

Many women experience difficulties reaching orgasm either with a partner or while masturbating. Many women have never learned through self-exploration how to bring themselves to orgasm, because of their belief that society disapproves of females touching and stimulating their bodies. More than half of American women don't climax all the time or at all during intercourse. Ten to fifteen percent of women have never had an orgasm, not even through masturbation, and another third orgasm only occasionally. This is often because American culture doesn't encourage females to lose their sexual inhibitions during their youth or to practice having orgasms.

Sometimes it's a matter of not knowing what an orgasm is all about. Studies have found that a few women, who claim to be anorgasmic (unable to experience climax), have physiological data that tells another story. These women do not perceive their bodies' signs of sexual climax as being an orgasm. These women have expectations regarding orgasm that are not met, and therefore, they don't identify orgasm when it occurs. Then there are women who have the complete opposite problem, who think they are having an orgasm but really aren't.

Some reasons you may not be reaching orgasm could include

1. You're thinking too much instead of enjoying the moment. You're wondering what your partner thinks of you, whether the two of you are moving well together, and if you're doing it "right." You need to get out of your head and let go!

2. You, and/or your partner, rush into sex, not giving yourself enough time to get fully aroused and to build to a climax. In many such cases, he gets off before you and, worse yet, may leave you hanging.

3. You are afraid that you won't orgasm, so you don't even bother trying and end up completely repressing your sexual response. Madison, a 20-year-old self-described sex kitten, exemplifies this point for us: "The first time I had sex, Thad and I were going at it for like a half hour before he asked me if I'd come. I looked at him, totally surprised, then explained to him that I didn't expect to orgasm since I'd read in *Cosmo* that only 10 percent of women

orgasm the first time they have sex. Maybe if I hadn't read that, I would've been a part of that 10 percent!"

4. You've always thought of sex as something dirty or something that you shouldn't enjoy. This guilt is getting in the way of you truly enjoying your sexual moments.

5. You're afraid that if your partner concentrates too much on your pleasure, you'll feel too much pressure to come and will freeze up.

6. You and your partner are trying too hard to have a simultaneous orgasm.

7. You're conflicted about your relationship with your partner or you're angry with your partner.

8. You need more direct stimulation of your clitoris or G-spot.

Some women, for whatever reason, do not experience orgasm on all or many occasions of sexual activity, but still report that they enjoy their sexual relationship and don't regard themselves as having a sexual problem. The extent to which a woman and/or her partner view her anorgasmia as a problem depends on his and/or her expectations. About 90 percent of women with anorgasmia overcome the disorder once they've learned to pleasure themselves and enjoy their sexual sensations. If you're suffering from anorgasmia, here are things you can do to overcome this condition:

1. Stimulate your clitoris during lovemaking or have your partner stimulate it for you. If he doesn't know where it is, show and tell!

2. Don't be bashful in telling your partner what you want. Sometimes people just need some instruction. And your lover will love it, because an active and excited partner can be very arousing.

3. Take the time to pleasure yourself without your partner. Masturbate! Fantasize!

4. Explore your G-spot. This could be a means to have an orgasm.

5. Try positions where you're going to get maximum pleasure, like the woman-on-top position.

6. Strengthen your PC muscle. Use of voluntary muscle contractions can increase the levels of your sexual sensations.

7. Focus on sensations rather than thoughts.

8. Examine your body with a mirror. Get to know your genitalia and make friends with it.

9. Don't look at masturbation or sex with a partner as goal-oriented. Great sex doesn't necessarily mean having an orgasm.

10. Use a vibrator. Have your partner use a vibrator on you.

CAN MEN BE MULTI-ORGASMIC?

Yes, it is possible! There are men out there who are able to separate their orgasmic contractions from their ejaculations, experiencing contractions that retreat a split second before full ejaculation, and then work toward orgasm again. It has been documented that some men can have anywhere from two to sixteen orgasms during a single sex session, with most multi-orgasmic guys averaging four orgasms per session. For some of these men, ejaculation occurs more than once during this time period as well.

After ejaculation, a man has a short resting period—a "refractory period." It is this period of time that forces a guy to rest up a little bit and even to lose his erection. With practice and control, however, most men can extend their sexual cycles and enjoy several mini-orgasms before a final climax. (This is sometimes achieved more easily by squeezing the tip of the penis before ejaculation.) All of this usually takes weeks to months of training, during which a man becomes familiar with the sensations that occur right before that "moment of ejaculatory inevitability," and by practicing pelvic-muscle exercises on a daily basis.

A small percentage of men seemingly lack a refractory period and are "naturally multi-orgasmic." One 24-year-old Energizer Sex Bunny I know, Brooks, is living proof of multi-orgasmic men (though his ability usually involves alcohol): "The multiple orgasm thing almost always occurs after I have been drinking, and it also occurs the first couple times I have intercourse with a woman. It must have to do with my excitement level and the intensity of the moment—I can just keep on going and going. Other than those situations, I must say it is rather difficult to achieve multiple orgasms."

Most men who experience multiple orgasms will ejaculate only once. It is even possible for a man to feel orgasmic sensations after ejaculation or to have a series of mini-orgasms that climax with ejaculation. Certain men, who are able to suppress their emission to feel these mini-orgasms, are usually also able to have an orgasm with ejaculation and still remain erect. (No worries, I go into this in more detail in Chapter 16.)

Orgasm as a Goal

"I feel a better sense of accomplishment if I make a woman consistently have orgasms. That's a bigger achievement than being able to sleep with a lot of girls or just get off myself. I don't want to just get on a girl and pound downtown. It's not necessarily that I have to have sex with a girl for an hour. It has to be high quality." So says the soon-to-be-much-sought-after, 21-year-old student Lenny.

Some people think that sex isn't good unless at least one of the two of you has an orgasm. Some people go even further than that, believing that multiple orgasms are what a couple should be striving for during sex. Both of those mindsets are unhealthy and detrimental to a sexual relationship. Sex can be out of this world, even without an orgasm, and multiple orgasms are like winning a sexual lotto. However, they're not to be used as a measure of a killer sex session or a lover's talents.

While obtaining one or more orgasms can be an intriguing challenge and endeavor, remember that this is the type of thinking that can do a lot of damage to your relationship and end up making the two of you unhappy. So if you find yourself becoming goal-oriented in bed on occasion, just remind yourself that only 29 percent of women *always* have an orgasm and that 75 percent of men *always* do. Interestingly enough, about 40 percent of both sexes are pleased with their sex lives. So a lot of people have realized that good sex isn't just about orgasm—it's about what you're *satisfied* with. Having that realization is in itself pretty heavenly.

Faking and Sex

To this day, popular magazines are still debating the ethical issue of faking orgasm. Is it okay? Wrong? An act of humanity? It's an issue that will never be laid to rest. Faking can be a good thing or it can eventually lead to your own sexual downfall.

By faking orgasm, you may feel you are being selfless and compassionate, sparing your partner's feelings, but in reality you are giving him or her a false sense of security as to their talents between the sheets and/or your own comfort. On the other hand, by faking, you're betraying your primal, sexual being, not letting your partner know all of your needs, how his or her techniques could be improved, and how sex, in general, could be a better experience for both of you. A 24-year-old construction worker, Jonny, would rather know than have a faker on his hands: "I can't stand a woman who thinks this is an acceptable form of boosting her man's self-esteem. I remember a famous quote on the issue: 'Men would rather be ineffective than lied to.' My sentiments exactly!"

Whether faking is saintly or sinful, by doing it, you're missing out on the opportunity to teach your partner how to make you climax. Sarah, a 25-year-old sex educator, backs my point: "Why fake? If it's someone you care about, then it seems dishonest. It's so important to communicate about what you like. A partner can't read your mind! And who says that you have to have an orgasm every time anyway? If you don't, that's okay. You shouldn't have to fake one just to make your partner feel better."

Lots of people fake orgasm. Sixty-one percent of women have faked a single orgasm and 63 percent have faked multiple orgasms. To make some of you female fakers feel better, there are some guys out there—about 18 percent of them—doing the exact same thing. (They can get away with it, too. Remember that orgasm doesn't necessarily equal ejaculation.)

Hunter, a 21-year-old alternative-music lover, is a classic case of a male faker:

> I had a girlfriend a couple of years ago and she would feel really insecure if I didn't orgasm soon—quick. So I would fake it on occasion because she would then feel that she was doing something right, and it made her think that I was great. I didn't feel badly doing it or even

guilty. I'd just throw on a good porn star face and give a little grunt.
I'd let my whole body shudder and then tell her I was going to come.
That's it.

Painfully easy to get away with, isn't it?

There is no surefire way to tell if your partner has had an orgasm.

WHY DO PEOPLE FAKE ORGASM?

So why are so many people faking it? Well, faking orgasm can be very functional. There are plenty of reasons why people fake, and perhaps rightfully so:

✳ Faking can allow you to get some sleep, as Miguel, a 23-year-old Latino heartthrob, admits: "I faked orgasm once because I was tired. I just kind of stopped like I was done. I don't feel guilty about it. Doing that allowed me to go to sleep."

✳ Faking can spare your partner's feelings. Lucy, a 24-year old who surfs the web to view photos of the hunks-of-hockey, exclaims:

Have I ever faked an orgasm?! With every partner! Normally, it was the case that my partner was not doing something right and I was getting tired of going through the motions and trying to make it work. So I just faked it to get the whole thing over with. . . . Never felt guilty about it. They always came, so I certainly didn't feel guilty about that. I felt like faking was an easy way to save their ego and avoid more attempts with the same results.

✳ Finally, what harm can be done if you're faking orgasm with a partner that you don't plan on sleeping with often or ever again? Shirl-dog, a 21-year-old fraternity boy, shares a time when faking came in especially handy for him:

One time when I was pledging, I was coming home from a house party with this girl. She'd been all over me all night, even had her hands down my pants. I was bombed and when I got home, I didn't know what I was doing. So we ended up going to my room. Big mistake. But anyway, I started having sex with this girl on these two beds I'd pushed together. As we were having sex, they started to come apart and I couldn't keep the mattresses together. So I had to stop and get up to fix the beds. When I turned the lights on, I saw her...and had sex with her for another minute and a half before I faked it. I pretty much lay there like I was done. She didn't know.

I'm not for or against faking. I'm rather neutral on the matter. Here's some advice for you, though: If you're going to fake, make sure that you can pull it off. Madison has a sorry story for us, showing why this is so important:

I'd had a sex-fest weekend with Dave and was riding him once again and just wanted to get it over with. Since he was a rather selfish lover, never seeming that concerned about whether or not I'd come, I thought there'd be no harm in me faking it to get things over with. Well, I forgot that Dave had been with quite a number of women and I'm sure had been with women who orgasmed or who had been great fakers. Having never had an orgasm myself, I was a terrible faker. He saw right through it and was not happy. I made a mental note to never pretend to orgasm again, or at least not until I knew what one was all about and could pull it off!

As you can see, orgasm is a very individual thing. It comes in as many different forms as there are people in this world. Each of us has our own formula for how we can have an orgasm, under what circumstances, and with whom. And remember, as long as you know your body and how to turn it on, using protection is not going to change this. You are in charge of your safer-sex orgasmic potential. As you will learn in later chapters, you can make this mind/body experience a healthy one, one that never fails to rock.

CHAPTER 3

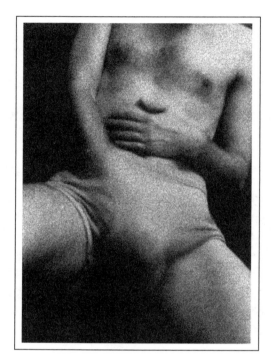

Solo
Sexplorations

Is masturbation normal?

Are there benefits to masturbating?

How do people "get off"?

Masturbation—that pumping state of solo, sexual frenzy with the hand or an object, during which you're stimulating your own genitals to produce sexual arousal. With lots of skill and just the right touch, you can send yourself on a roundtrip flight to ecstasy, soaring all the way to oblivion, almost any time and as many times as you want. What a trip!

Ready to book your ticket? Autoeroticism is the **safest kind of sex** you can have. It's quality time with yourself that not only enables you to understand your body's preferences as far as what feels good, but also teaches you how you become most effectively aroused. It helps you to safely develop the skills and techniques your body thrives on for the ultimate touch-your-body experience. Plus, making love to yourself helps you to develop sexual comfort and security with your body and sexuality and, in doing so, raises your self-esteem.

Before I continue singing the praises of self-stimulation, I must acknowledge that a lot of people, mostly women, are really uncomfortable dealing with it. I remember back in high school, when my friends and I would lightly broach the matter over lunch. One girl would always throw a hissy fit if we started talking about it because she felt that it was *too* much. Then, after each of us made a face and swore we'd never ever have the desire to touch ourselves in *that* way, we'd all conclude that masturbation was gross. Knowing what I know now about masturbation, I bet that at least half the girls in that group were masturbators.

I can't blame my lunchmates, though, for not spilling the beans on their self-pleasure practices. Masturbation is a very private thing and very much your own business. The real shame in all of the privacy, however, is that even if the girls had wanted to share, they were not given the discretion to do so. We're all expected to keep it secret.

I wish that our modern culture could be more mature about the subject of masturbation. Our media, religious groups, most parents, and even the government don't know how to handle the subject and so choose to oppose it or ignore it. Such negative thinking about self-stimulation is further fostered by the way society raises us to ignore our bodies' sexual urges and discourages us from self-discovery. Seems kind of silly since masturbation is such a good thing, really quite harmless. So why is our society like that?

A Brief History of Masturbation

Almost all societies disapprove of masturbation on some level that ranges from mild ridicule to severe punishment. American society, on the whole, has given masturbation a bad rap over the years, preaching that it is an evil, dirty, harmful behavior and a threat to the natural goal of sexuality—reproduction. Even now in the twenty-first century, we're still recovering from church teachings from the "old country" that called masturbation a "mortal and diabolical" sin; from doctors in the 1700s who linked masturbation to insanity; and from the field of psychiatry, which had even labeled masturbation as a type of nervous disorder (like epilepsy) at one point. Even the sexually liberal psychoanalyst Sigmund Freud regarded masturbation as harmful to the genitals and to one's psychosexual and moral development. With all of this kind of thinking over the years, it is no wonder that we still use the term "masturbation," which was derived from the Latin verb *masturbare,* meaning "to defile or disturb by hand," when referring to the act.

During the Victorian era, people viewed semen as an essential substance for a man's health and well-being, and one not to be wasted—a view still espoused by some groups, e.g., Taoists. Sylvester Graham (1794–1851) believed that by ejaculating, a man lowered his life force and exposed his body to disease and early death. Graham advised Victorians to use foods of unsifted wheat flour, like graham flour, to reduce their sexual desire. Hence, those famous Graham crackers we all know and love!

Societies have come up with plenty of far-out myths as a means of deterring young people from stimulating themselves. So in case you've heard them, know that there is no scientific basis for the myths that masturbation leads to acne, warts, hair on the palm, insanity, mental retardation, epilepsy, impotence, sterility, sexual perversion, poor physical health, physical deformities, blindness, deafness, or homosexuality. In addition, masturbation is *not* selfish or immature, you *cannot* become addicted to it, it is *not* harmful, and women do it too. Masturbation is not something to be ashamed of, nor is it something that is going to have harmful effects on your body or being.

With all of the above myths, it is no wonder that we live in a sexually dysfunctional society that can't handle masturbation. Many people have difficulties in their relationships, in becoming aroused, and in performing certain sexual acts because they are very inhibited about their sexuality, partly because they are not in tune with their sexual being and because they refrain from masturbating or feel guilty doing so.

The world would be such a happier place if more people took the time for self-exploration and pleasuring. Maybe it's the secret to world peace. I don't know. I do know, though, that if more people masturbated, fewer people would suffer from sexual dysfunctions and more people would be enjoying sex—solo or not—to its fullest.

Even if you don't like to masturbate or don't want to, you should embrace autoeroticism, for it doesn't need to be limited to sexual activity. Everyone is into self-pleasure in one way or another, so don't limit yourself to thinking that it's strictly sexual! Autoeroticism can be about enjoying life's simple pleasures—going for a run along the waterfront at sunrise, soaking in a hot tub, smelling fresh flowers, driving with the top down ... anything your body gets off on.

> Kellogg's Corn Flakes was originally marketed as a cure for masturbation.

Who Masturbates?

With all the myths and negative beliefs about masturbation that continually circulate through society, people can get the wrong impression about it, thinking that self-stimulation is an unhealthy activity that only the lonely find themselves doing. *Au contraire!* Lots of people masturbate, and it can have an enormous, positive impact on one's sexuality. Masturbation is even found in the animal kingdom, with animals like male red deer and female porcupines doing it. It is particularly common among primates, who have been seen either stimulating their genitals or rubbing them against objects. Even human male fetuses experience erections and stroke their penises while in the womb, and research has shown that human female fetuses experience vaginal lubrication while in utero, perhaps as a result of arousal.

Even before we're born, we're sexually functioning beings, discovering our own sexuality.

Sarah remembers masturbating at an early age:

> I have vivid memories of masturbating to orgasm when I was very young—less than 5 years old. In fact, I was still in a bed that had sides on it to protect me from rolling out and falling on the floor! Of course, I didn't understand what it was at that point. I just knew that it would feel really good, then get very intense and then I would just know to stop because the sensations would go away. I was never scolded, but somehow I knew this was something to do in private! I've continued masturbating since then, although how often varies quite a lot. I might go weeks without doing it and then other times it might be a daily occurrence.

Geoffrey, a 23-year-old writer, recalls joining the ranks at a slightly later age, discovering masturbation upon reaching puberty:

> I discovered masturbation when I was 11 or 12 years old. I had my first orgasm by accident one night when I rolled over on my erection. So that's how I kept doing it. I didn't realize I could use my hand for a while—two years. Now I masturbate on average seven to ten times a week. It's almost like any other bodily function. It varies with other things, like if I'm under a lot of stress. I probably do it a lot because I've always been in major, monogamous relationships, but whether or not I'm in a relationship has never affected my habits.

The reality is that many people have found that masturbation is an ideal outlet for expressing and satisfying sexual needs. Almost all men and a majority of women (82 percent) masturbate to orgasm at least a few times during their lives.

Masturbation Gender Differences

Of the men and women who do masturbate, men tend to masturbate more often than women, ranging from one time a month to two to three times per day. This is really too bad for the ladies, since masturbation has been found to be the most reliable of all forms of sexual activity for producing orgasm.

Knowing this, it's a wonder that many women begin masturbating at an older age, often *after* they've started having sexual intercourse. Female masturbators also masturbate more often while in a relationship. This is especially interesting if you consider that young men usually masturbate *less* if they are in a relationship.

Why less solo time for the men? There's no surefire answer, but Frodo, a 25-year-old self-described horny poet, takes a stab at explaining this interesting correlation: "When it comes to masturbating, it depends on if I'm in a relationship. I don't think I ever have masturbated while in a relationship. I think of it as something you use when you need to, when you haven't had anything in a long time."

Eighty percent of men and 60 percent of women always or usually have an orgasm during masturbation.

Chances are, by the time you've reached young adulthood, you've already done a fair share of self-exploration. Whether you're a "masterbator" or are self-pleasuring for the first time, you may want to practice some of the following techniques. In setting the mood, refer back to Step 1 of the Body-Image Exercise and/or the date with yourself tips in Chapter 1.

FEMALE MASTURBATION EXERCISES

1. Focus your attention on manipulating your clitoris and inner lips (the most common way a female masturbates), preferably using lubricant. Rub your clit in an up/down or circular motion, either lightly or with pressure. The amount of clitoral stimulation that you can handle and enjoy may vary from time to time. Some women find direct stimulation too intense and prefer rubbing the side of the clitoris, while others like their clitoris to be the focus of attention and may work it 'til it goes numb with pleasure.

2. While doing this, rub and squeeze your thighs together for added pressure and stimulation, perhaps while massaging your pubic area.

3. Play with your inner lips by stroking them or tugging at them. Since your clitoris and inner lips are connected, any direct or indirect stimulation to the inner lips can be sexually exciting. A

combination of any of these methods may be used at the same time.

4. Insert one or more fingers into your vagina with a thrusting or circular motion. This can be wildly intense if done at the same time as you play with your clitoris.

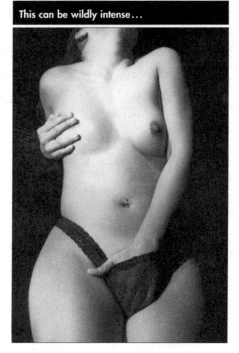

This can be wildly intense...

5. If you're a crafty female masturbator, you'll make sure that the rest of your body parts aren't ignored. Tweak or rub your nipples, or cup and massage your breasts as you're getting off. Some women also find that sexual feelings may be heightened further during masturbation by contracting the anal muscles and/or inserting a finger or sex toy into the rectum. No matter what the method, many women who become comfortable with their bodies through masturbation can orgasm in as little as four minutes!

6. As far as other penetration methods go, you may insert fingers, dildos, ice cubes, popsicle sticks, etc. No matter what the method or sex toy involved, if you do it effectively, you may be the lucky person who experiences over twenty-five consecutive orgasms while performing a masturbatory technique!

7. Use a stream of water to massage your clitoris, or press your clitoris against an object, like a pillow. Other methods may include a handheld shower massage, jets in a pool or hot tub, vibrators....

Taking Matters into Her Own Hands

Studies have shown that the frequency of masturbation activity increases for most women during menstruation, while the amount of intercourse they have decreases.

MALE MASTURBATION EXERCISES

1. Arm yourself with lubricant. A lot of guys like to go to town with lube, e.g., soap suds or baby oil, and lather up their prized possession beforehand.

2. Circle your hand around your penis and move it up and down your shaft, making the motion more and more vigorous as you continue.

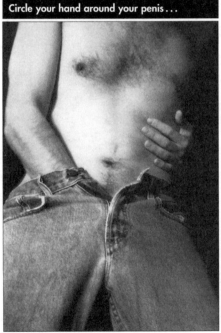

Circle your hand around your penis...

3. Concentrate on the head—stroking the glans and frenulum. You may prefer using only light touches on the tip, or strong, gripping movements across the entire penis.

4. Try pulling at the skin of the scrotal sac, varying degrees of pressure on the shaft, inserting a finger into the rectum, rolling your penis against your body.

5. Massage the anus, scrotum, testicles, nipples, and your whole body. Contract the anal muscles, perhaps even using a sex toy for added stimulation. Note that you may reach orgasm in as little as one or two minutes.

✳ **Why Masturbate?** ✳

Perhaps you don't think that sexual fulfillment, self-pleasuring, and the chance to get in touch with your sexual being are enough reason to get off? Perhaps, then, one of the following reasons will float your boat. Masturbation is great because:

- It's absolute, 100-percent-safe sex.

- You can totally avoid pregnancy and sexually transmitted infections, including HIV.

- For ladies, it helps to keep your vagina lubricated and builds resistance to yeast infections.

- It's a super form of stress reduction and it relieves sexual tension.

- It's a means of endorphin release—it can make you smile.

- Women may overcome premenstrual tension and other physical conditions, like cramps, that are associated with their menstrual cycles.

- It leads to relaxed sleeping conditions.

- It builds stronger pelvic muscles.

- For men, it builds resistance to prostate gland infection.

- It's an excellent cardiovascular workout.

- It increases your sexual awareness.

- It can be done when no partner is available.

- It's the exploration of various kinds of self-stimulation, especially the sensations and pleasures that are maximally satisfying for you.

- It's empowering!

- It allows you to participate in sex more frequently than you can with a partner.

- It helps you to think more positively about your genitalia.

- It enhances your sex life.

* You have longer periods of arousal and near-orgasm than you would with a partner.

* More intense orgasms result.

* You want to become a better lover. (Women, pay special attention here. Men have told me that their better lovers have been the females who've masturbated.) Mallory, a 24-year-old artist, agrees: "Masturbation is the way to go to have better sex with your partner. When you know how to stimulate yourself, then you can show a guy how to do it and do it well. Guys need to learn stuff like that from girls. They want to. It totally helps!"

There is no such thing as too much masturbating, unless you do it to the point of causing physical harm, e.g., rubbing yourself sore repeatedly. You can do it to your heart's content, and there is nothing wrong with you for it. Men should learn to control ejaculation and not get off too quickly while playing with themselves, since this can help them to make love longer when with a partner. Self-pleasuring only requires having the space, time, and privacy for having fun with yourself. So play away!

If you're still hesitating about masturbating, consider it in a different light—it's the most reliable form of self-entertainment that you can count on using, within reasonable limits, anytime and anywhere. For instance, say you're stranded on a deserted island all by yourself, with no chance of rescue anytime soon—a "Gilligan's Island" sort of scenario. You've exhausted all of the island entertainment, like gathering coconuts for dinner or swimming in the lagoon. You're looking for something to do and have only yourself to rely on. On top of that, you haven't fooled around in *so* long and aren't into the whole bestiality thing as an alternative. What can you do?

Masturbate! Can you think of a better self-involved thing to do that could last up to a couple of hours? All you need is a little bit of hand motion and you're in business! I challenge you to come up with a better, more exhilarating way to easily, enjoyably pass solo time on that little island and turn it into paradise.

You also might want to check out Betty Dodson's book, *Sex for One: The Joy of Selfloving.* It's a great book for becoming "sex-positive" [her term] in general and comfortable with masturbation specifically.

CHAPTER 4

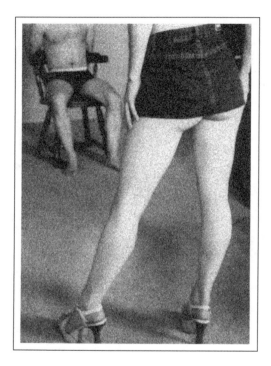

You Always
Can in
Fantasyland

How do men's and women's sexual fantasies differ?

How can fantasy enhance your sex life?

Fantasy is a normal and healthy means of self-stimulation to heighten sexual experience and enjoyment. Fantasy is your mind's own private photo album or movie reel of erotic objects or acts that put the beat in your libido. During fantasy, you become your own romance screenwriter or XXX-rated film director, creating visual imagery that's sexually exciting to you, like imagining his bobbing, madly thrusting head between your thighs. Fantasy can also be a sexually charged longing or past turn-on, such as remembering the first time you felt her damp, satin underwear as your fingers fumbled their way into her slippery, inviting vagina.

One of the best things about fantasy is that no physical exertion needs to be involved. Your mind does all of the work! Fantasy can be a substitute for sex; it can lead to sex; it can add spice to your sex life; and when you act it out, it can take you and your partner to uncharted sexual territory. Best yet, it's safe sex and is a dependable way of eroticizing safer sex. In addition, fantasy is great because it can be a private way of enjoying thoughts that turn you on, but that you are not able to or would not wish to act out in reality.

Who Fantasizes?

People often get weirded out when it comes to fantasy—who me do it? —No way! Fantasy is one of those topics people stay away from for fear that they'll be ostracized if they admit to actually doing it. On the occasion that it does come up in conversation, people recoil from the subject because they worry that others will find them strange or perverted if it's found out that they fantasize and, even more so, what they fantasize about.

This standoffish attitude toward fantasy is certainly understandable because it is such a private thing, one that's hard to openly discuss. It's not that anybody necessarily *has* to talk about their fantasies and make them publicly known. One of the best things about your fantasies is that they are your own, so personal that they are nobody else's business. Yet society has stigmatized fantasy so much that these sensual, erotic, titillating thoughts do not always get the credit they deserve.

The downside of fantasy being a rather hush-hush topic is that a lot of people are suffering sexually because of it. Case in point—15 percent of men and women try to repress the feelings of arousal they have when they have sexual fantasies and thoughts since they consider those natural mental images to be a negative thing. Fantasy is seen as forbidden and sinful and, hence, triggers guilt, shame, anxiety, and uneasiness. Consequently, up to one quarter of Americans feel great guilt about the sexual fantasies they have *during* sex, and are more likely than people who don't have this guilt to feel that such thoughts are immoral, uncommon, abnormal, and socially unacceptable.

So with all of these people out there fearful of fantasy, who fantasizes? While most people blush upon hearing the word "fantasy" and pretend that they don't do it, 84 percent of men and 82 percent of women report fantasizing at least some of the time, and both sexes report that positive feelings accompany sexual arousal and fantasy.

Such a healthy, positive ability to fantasize leads to people engaging in sexual intercourse much more frequently than individuals who don't fantasize, maybe because they are also more likely to use fantasy to enhance sex. Men and women who use fantasy and autoerotic materials (e.g., pornography, sex toys) are also those who seek out the most sex with their partners and who find the greatest number of other sexual experiences and practices appealing. Furthermore, fantasizers tend to be the people who are the most interested in sex and who are the most sexually active.

Benefits of Fantasy

✳   It's a form of safe sex.

✳   It can help you get aroused and hard, or wet.

✳   It can help you reach orgasm—push you over the edge!

✳   You can fantasize whenever, wherever you want to.

✳   You can revisit your fantasies whenever you want to.

✳   It can help you get through a sex session with somebody you do not find desirable.

* It is an inexpensive and effective sexual enhancer.

* It can help you overcome your anxieties and hesitations about sex and become more sexually confident.

* It acts as a way to explore new sexual outlets.

* It can bolster your self-image, making you feel sexual, attractive, powerful, loved, and desired.

Your fantasies don't even have to be terribly exciting to get you going or to be enjoyable. They don't need to be hard-core or graphic to be good fantasies. Sometimes, just thinking of yourself as a much-adored superstar is the simplest and best kind of fantasy.

Sarah describes the fantasies that cross her mind:

> My fantasies tend to be on the boring side . . . no elaborate scenes that I act out or detailed scenarios. In fact, there are rarely faces involved. Instead, my fantasies tend to be around specific sexual acts. If I saw something in a movie that looked interesting, then I will envision myself doing that particular thing, but not with anyone in particular. And they tend to be quite selfish. I am the center of the fantasy and usually everything is being done to me!

Differences Between Male and Female Fantasies

Men and women are always wondering what the other sex fantasizes about—what turns them on or gets them off, and who they're fantasizing about. While most people expect major differences between the two, the truth is that male and female fantasies aren't too different from one another. The most common fantasies for both males and females involve having a threesome (whatever the combination) and using a video camera—*action!* Both sexes also fantasize about current partners, reliving past experiences, and oral sex.

Naturally, though, there are some gender differences when it comes to fantasy. Ever since Alfred Kinsey's revolutionary sex study in 1948, a number of researchers like Gagnon and Simon and Ellis and Symons have been reporting interesting findings about sexual fantasy. Women tend to fantasize more about new lovemaking positions, making love in exotic/romantic places, being forced to have sex, bondage, being found irresistible by males, sex with a new partner, and doing something "wicked." Male fantasies include sensual, nongenital lovemaking (without the penis or vagina!), being made love to, orgies, voyeurism, and being aggressive or dominant during sex.

FEMALE FANTASIES

Female sexual fantasies are more likely than male fantasies to contain familiar partners and to include descriptions of the context *(greeting him in only a trench coat after months of separation),* setting *(at the airport),* and feelings associated with the sexual encounter *(this tigress is all about lust and longing).* Their fantasized sexual partners are typically guys they are or have been romantically or sexually involved with.

Their fantasies have been found to contain more affection, love, passion, and commitment, focusing on their imagined partner's personal *(he's funny)* or emotional *(he's sensitive)* characteristics. They are also more likely to emphasize themes of tenderness and emotionality *(running his fingers through her hair as he tells her what a fool he was for breaking her heart to go back to his ex-girlfriend).*

Some studies have shown that women are more likely than men to be only emotionally, rather than physically, aroused by their sexual fantasies. Yet there are plenty of women who get sexually charged and physically aroused from their fantasies, with a few women lucky enough to obtain orgasm through fantasy alone!

It has also been documented that female fantasies are much more likely than men's to build s-l-o-w-l-y to explicitly sexual activity. Women fantasize more about their own attractiveness to men *(she has the most beautiful body he's ever seen)* and the emotional context of the sexual activity that is exciting them *(she's the only woman he'll ever need).* More often than not, they're fantasizing that they're being submissive *(I'm all yours. Play with me).* On the whole, female sexual fantasies tend to be more contextual, emotional, intimate, and passive.

Sexually experienced women are more likely than virgins to have explicit sexual fantasies.

MALE FANTASIES

Men are more likely to have sexual fantasies and to be physically aroused by their sexual thoughts than women. They are more than twice as likely as women to report having sexual fantasies and becoming aroused at least once a day. They're also twice as likely as females to fantasize about having a greater number of different partners during the course of an average day.

A guy is also more likely to have a sexual fantasy about someone whom he simply would like to have sex with, such as that hot chick he always sees working out at the gym, than about someone he is or has been sexually or romantically involved with. Byron, for example, has fantasies involving his ideal woman: "Lots of things go through my mind when I masturbate—a potential woman versus any particular woman per se. I have this image of an ideal woman. I think of her as a possible wife or lover, but that's more of a fantasy since she's not real, just an ideal."

A lot of women get insecure about the fact that men think about other women when they fantasize. This is understandable, since we all don't look like *Penthouse* Pets, the pretty, raven-haired intern he drools over, or your bombshell best friend he's always hinting at having join in for a threesome. Yet not all men daydream about other women all of the time, like Jake, a 25-year-old researcher, who shares: "I fantasize about my partner because she drives me crazy. I think about her all the time!"

Men are also more likely to have specifically sexual dreams while they sleep. His sexual fantasies are much more likely than a female's fantasy to include specific sexual acts *(doing her doggie style),* sexual organs *(her cappuccino-colored, erect nipples),* and a greater variety of visual content, like having a clear image of the genital features of their fantasy partner *(her glistening vaginal opening).* Male fantasies focus on female bodies *(butts, breasts, hips),* the actual sexual activity they're envisioning *(orgy with this month's* Playboy *Bunnies),* and especially the responses of their fantasized partner *(heavy panting).* Male fantasies are more likely to focus on minute details of their partner's physical appearance and to involve strangers, multiple partners, or anonymous partners.

Men also like to see themselves in their own fantasies as being dominant. When he fantasizes, *he is He-man.* Men are more likely than women to view others as the objects of their sexual desires instead of being the object of desire. Geoffrey almost can't believe it himself that he always needs to be thinking of a woman in order to get off: "I have to have a woman to focus on, an object of fantasy. This is going to sound weird, but if I don't have a clear idea of someone in mind, I won't come. I have to concentrate. It's funny because it's a solitary activity, yet still directed toward the other person."

Men are twice as likely as women to experience an externally provoked sexual fantasy, meaning one that's a response to something they've heard, read, or seen in the environment. So looking at magazines, books, or videos with nudity is usually enough to get a guy going. In summary, male sexual fantasies tend to take place more frequently and tend to be more visual, specifically sexual, promiscuous, and active.

The Role Fantasy Plays in Masturbation

Fantasy can add just the right flavor to any masturbation activity. To go through the physical motions of turning yourself on is one thing, but opening your mind to erotic fantasies can take playing with yourself to a whole new dimension.

More men (87 percent) than women (69 percent) report having had sexual fantasies during masturbation. Men usually fantasize about someone they know, while women fantasize about a current partner or interest. Geoffrey explains that his fantasy girls are always women he somehow knows:

> I can't successfully fantasize about a woman with whom I've never had any sort of contact. For example, Nicole Kidman is a beautiful woman, but I could never masturbate thinking of her because I've never talked to her. I have nothing on which to base that she might be attracted to me. If I were to meet her on the street and come away thinking she disliked me or was indifferent, it would still be difficult. The hook-up has to be possible.

Women who report having frequent sexual fantasies while masturbating become sexually aroused with greater intensity than do women who use masturbation fantasy less frequently. Most people who have fantasies during masturbation envision giving or receiving oral sex. Usually, the setting is a romantic one. At times, the fantasy involves sexual power or irresistibility—being forced to or forcing someone to have sex. **Note:** This does not at all mean that a person wants to actually have forced sex!

Petra, a 24-year-old athletic graduate student, has a really racy fantasy when she's going at it solo:

What puts me over the edge every time lately when I'm masturbating is imagining myself as a dancer at a club. I'm on stage with another chick and the whole place is FILLED with men. The other woman and I are going at it on stage and the men have to be held back from the stage by bouncers. They are all yelling for us to keep going. Then, two more women come out and they both hold my legs down. One of them starts using a vibrator on my clit. The men in the club are going crazy, yelling, throwing money at us. She keeps the vibrator on my clit and the club director comes on stage. He says, "Come on, this is what you're here for! You'd better come now or you won't get paid! All these men are here for you! Stick that pussy up in the air and come for us now!!" That does it and I enter the wonderful world of orgasm. . . .

Fantasizing about the Same Sex

Even if you are heterosexual, your sex drive may find the thought of hooking up with your own gender very erotic—which is perfectly okay. If you find yourself enjoying a fantasy involving a partner of your own sex, it doesn't necessarily mean that you're gay or bisexual. It's just that the idea of it turns you on. Fantasies don't always represent unconscious desires.

Mason explains that sometimes she finds fantasizing about women more arousing:

Though I would never want to hook up with another woman, I fantasize about another girl messing around with me on occasion. It's one of those lipstick lesbian fantasies and almost always it's her doing something to me—going down on me, feeling me out, obeying me. . . . Sometimes it's a lot more arousing than fantasizing about a guy, probably because it's sort of taboo. Given an actual opportunity to hook up with a female, I'd never do it. The thought of that actually turns me off. But your fantasies are your own thing. You can make anything happen or not.

The Kinsey Scale

Your sexual orientation describes who you are sexually and romantically attracted to, whom you lust after and love. In the 1940s, biologist Alfred Kinsey developed the Kinsey Scale for Sexual Orientation, a seven-point scale depicting sexual attraction as a continuum. This scale challenged the notion that your attraction and sexual identity, how you think of yourself in terms of your sexual orientation, are black and white—that you're either homosexual or heterosexual. The Kinsey scale offers gray, arguing that most people aren't strictly heterosexual or homosexual, and that a person's place on the scale can change over time. If you're at…

The Kinsey scale

```
   |     |     |     |     |     |     |
   0     1     2     3     4     5     6
```

Zero: You've never had a homosexual thought, fantasy, or experience. You're exclusively heterosexual and only attracted to, desire, fantasize about, and have sex with the opposite sex.

One: You're predominantly heterosexual with slight homosexual tendencies. You may think of someone of the same sex and have fantasies and fleeting desires.

Two: You're bisexual with substantial homosexual experience, but leaning toward heterosexuality. You have had sexual contact with your gender.

Three: You're bisexual—attracted to both sexes.

Four: You're bisexual with substantial heterosexual experience but leaning toward homosexuality. You have had sexual contact with the other gender.

Five: You're predominantly homosexual with the occasional heterosexual tendency. You may think of someone of the opposite sex and have fantasies and fleeting desires.

Six: You're strictly homosexual and all about people of the same sex. You've never had a heterosexual thought, fantasy, or experience.

So where do you fit into the scale? Most people fall between one and two. I really like this scale because it takes on all these silly labels our society loves and it captures your erotic potential, normalizing it and making it okay because it is okay. It also helps to explain why some of your thoughts, fantasies, and desires might not always align themselves with your sexual identity or orientation.

Resources

If you're wondering whether you're gay, straight, or bisexual, or if you've determined that you're gay or lesbian and are looking for support in coming to terms with that realization or breaking the news to others, contact the following organization:

Gay and Lesbian National Hotline: (888) THE-GLNH or www.glnh.org

What to Do When One Becomes Two

Now that we've covered the basics about your sexual self,

Part II of the book takes a look at what happens when you

involve someone else in your sex life. This is where being

informed about safer sex really starts to matter.

CHAPTER 5

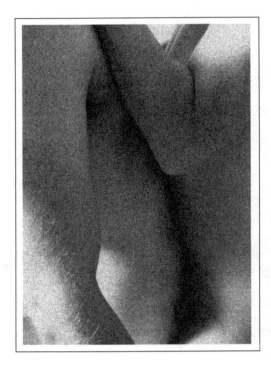

Navigating Your Love Life

What do people find attractive?

How can you attract somebody?

What's it like to be in love?

Who cheats?

What should you consider in having a threesome?

How do you know if you've found "The One"?

Attraction

Whether or not we're aware of it, many of our daily thoughts and activities revolve around concerns about being attractive, about impressing others with our looks, and about image. Should I shower this morning in case I run into that hottie I've been digging or should I sleep in? Can I get away with no makeup today? Do I need to start lifting weights? Should I go on a diet?

THE BIOLOGY OF BEAUTY

What look do most people go for? What do people find attractive about the opposite sex? Even scientists have tried to figure out what goes into sex appeal for males and females. Not surprisingly, the research reveals that male attractiveness is marked by outward signs of maturity, health, and dominance. Female markers of beauty signal youthfulness and an abundance of reproductive hormones. Even if you're not seeking to procreate with your mate, biology may influence what you find attractive. Certain characteristics show that he has good genes and has promise as a provider for his offspring, and that she is fertile and of childbearing age. Overall, humans are said to love symmetry, favoring average-looking features over unusual ones, most likely because unusual characteristics would be more likely to carry harmful genetic mutations. There's growing research about what makes a human attractive—what makes for the ideal male or female. While that research is interesting, it's not really relevant for those of us striving to love ourselves the way we are. Besides, there's another important factor in beauty that deserves much more attention—positive attitude.

> When it comes to sexual relationships, both men and women find a partner's physical characteristics to be more important than their personal characteristics. This is not the case, however, in long-term romantic relationships.

WHAT REAL BEAUTY IS ALL ABOUT

Positive Attitude

No matter what you look like, no matter what your size is, positive attitude ("'tude") is where it's at: a mix of healthy self-esteem, good energy, and boldness. Positive attitude is very attractive; it helps you to succeed. Positive attitude is letting everyone else know that you believe in yourself, and I don't mean in a cocky or bitchy kind of way. You have to be careful about the type of positive attitude you project because being too sure of yourself can come across as being full of yourself. Having an overblown ego is such a turn-off, plus it indicates that you probably have an inferiority complex or insecurity issues more than anything. That's very unattractive.

Positive attitude is your best friend when you're out on the town. It is what attracts others to you, what helps you work the scene and come out on top. Positive attitude is what helps you play the "mating game."

When I think of famous people with 'tude who are sexy, a number of stars come to mind: Prince, Blondie's Debbie Harry, Will Smith, Halle Berry, Jimmy Fallon.... These people are attractive because the attitude they have is rooted in their true beauty—their ability to tap into their creative talents, to be funny, to express themselves, to carry themselves with dignity and grace, to be sexy.

Obviously, I think that these stars have it going on, and I mention them here only to give you examples of people with great positive attitude because most of you don't know Emma, one of my best friends in the world, who has the best positive attitude going, as you can see from this e-mail she recently sent me:

> Let's go out and drink light beer and make each other laugh and wink at random people and flirt and kiss cheeks and laugh and dance with our arms high in the air and smoke cigars sensually and show leg

"unintentionally" and then dance with the hottest guys because we can. You know how people complain about the dating scene and say how they're tired of "playing the game"? Well—let me just tell you the galldarn honest truth: I LOVE the GAME.

It's fun. If you go out with the right attitude, a girl can get any guy she wants. You just have to have attitude and play yourself off perfectly. It's a BLAST! It's practically an ART FORM, you know? So next time you hear someone talking about the "games" men and women play and how they are just so frustrated with it, just remember: I'd rather be playing games than sitting on my big ass bored at home, so ROLL THE DICE, BABY.

True attitude is feeling secure with who you are and what you're all about. You have to be confident in yourself, believe in yourself. Attitude is about your inner beauty making your outer beauty shine. Believe me, other people, like Lenny, see it:

Just plain looks don't turn me on. Hot chicks don't turn me on, maybe because I think I won't like their personality because they're so into their looks, too into themselves.

I like attitude in a girl's demeanor. Her smile. The way she laughs… that's an indication of how she is as a person and that's more attractive…. A certain something about her—a certain characteristic that's seen in her attitude. That's what makes it become a long-term attraction versus a short-term, "Oh yeah, she's really hot!"

Positive attitude is believing that you're a superstar!! Do it right and 'tude is sexy.

Finding a Partner

Now that you're armed with a better sense of how to attract others, before you go on the man or woman hunt, you have to know what you're looking for. For most of us, this is already rather defined. First, unless we do something unusual, like move across country, we mainly associate with people who share our geographic locale and social circles. We tend to go for people who are not only similar to us in age, race, and education, but who share our attitudes and beliefs as well. We like those who have similar outlooks on life, who prefer similar activities, and who like the same kinds of people we do. Such preferences for individuals who share our values and beliefs allow for smooth and rewarding interactions, which always make life easier. So while opposites may attract on occasion, they seldom last.

RIGHT UNDER YOUR NOSE

Chances are your potential partner already shares your social network. You are more likely to know your partner in a context, such as school or work, and you could very well be friends already. If this partner-to-be of yours is of the same social background, it is unlikely that the two of you will be able to define your relationship as a short-term, sexual one. It's harder to have sex with people in your social circle and then just forget about it. There are greater investments and costs involved than if you found someone outside of your social network. So if things ever develop with someone in your social network, be cautious about moving too quickly toward sex, because misunderstandings could have a personal cost to you and your posse!

PICK-UP TIPS

Whether you're attracted to someone in your social network or want to hit the pick-up scene, there are several things you should keep in mind to encourage Cupid to strike. So my friend Veronica, a 25-year-old entrepreneur and accomplished pick-up artist, and I came up with this list of sure-fire ways to attract hotties!

   ∗   **Look your best**. Regardless of how you typically present yourself, before you go out, work your best look to a T, taking care to show your best features. Not only will this make you more attractive, but you'll go out feeling confident and better about yourself.

   ∗   **Use eye contact**. It's the most common initial sexual advance since it reveals a sparked interest, and since it is so common, the person you're desiring will most likely not mistake this nonverbal invitation. Eye contact makes it easier for somebody to respond to you. So if you've been eyeing somebody across the room, hold their gaze longer than you normally would, to show your interest. Give a demure look, but don't overdo it! Stares get scary, as Veronica explains: "I can flirt like a champ. Eye contact is the number-one flirting technique I can think of. . . subtle, but also obvious. It's all about timing. Look over and catch their smile, hold their gaze and smile for a second longer than you usually would, look away, look back and for a little longer this time, but not so long that it looks like you're staring."

If you're already engaged in conversation with the person, look at him or her directly. Focus all of your attention on that person and not on the person behind his shoulder or on the scuff on her shoe.

✳ **Smile.** This sends the message that you find the person attractive and that you'd like to continue the conversation. Plus, it's an indication that you're friendly and having a good time.

✳ **Carry yourself confidently.** Stand straight and don't slouch.

✳ **Step in toward the person.** This sends the signal that you'd like to get closer. You're allowing the person into your personal space, which in our society is a sign that you feel a certain level of comfort and with liking for the individual.

Note: Do a breath check first. Nothing can kill a move like this faster than bad breath. Not your problem? Usually, it's the people who have *halitosis* (chronic bad breath) who are the least aware of having it.

✳ **Make room for the person.** Gesture for him to sit down next to you, or move over so that she has standing space. Both of these actions let the person know that you'd like to talk a bit more. Furthermore, lean in when the person says something. This shows that you're actively listening to what they have to say and that you're interested in it. Or pretend you didn't hear something that was just said. That way one or both of you may have to move closer to hear something said a second time.

* **Give little, light touches.** "Accidentally" touch his hand or brush against her arm when you're excited about something you're talking about. Be subtle with these touches, not pushy.

* While in conversation, **ask specific, open-ended questions**, like, "So how did you get into this place if you're only 19?" instead of a yes/no question like, "Do you come here often?" This demonstrates that you're interested in what the person has to say and keeps the conversation alive. Make sure to also pause in between sentences. This shows that you're very relaxed and sure of yourself.

* **Give sincere compliments.** Don't tell somebody they have nice eyes or a great smile unless you mean it. Plus, try to give a compliment that they're not as likely to have heard. This lets the person know that you've been paying attention.

* **Whisper.** Dropping your voice forces the person you're talking to to lean in.

* **Be polite.** Use "please" and "thank you." Polite terminology is sadly becoming a thing of the past. Not enough people use it often enough. Therefore, you will seem that much more classy and attractive for being polite.

* **Do something to stand out.** With everyone these days trying to look like Jennifer Aniston or a male model from Abercrombie and Fitch, wear, bring, or carry something out of the ordinary when you go out, e.g., a friend of mine took a mini-football to a party, giving guys the perfect excuse to talk to her.

Relationships

I have decided that men are like disposable razors. They make you look and feel great at first, but after a while they either get dull or they nick you and it's time to throw them away and get a new one. Virtual BICS with dicks.

A very jaded friend of mine once e-mailed me this comment, frustrated with her love life. I think all of us—men and women—have had our moments when we have been fed up with our love lives and the people we're coming across, "shaving" with, and eventually disposing of.

We're all such razors. A partner can make you feel oh-so-smooth. Then one day, you discover that that razor of yours has gotten dull, or it cuts you, and you don't feel so sleek anymore. We're all too disposable.

I think that relationships are the hardest sexuality topic to tackle. They're subjective, individual, and emotionally laden, and it's difficult to acknowledge that while relationships can give us the best of times, they can also bring us the worst.

I feel bad not giving this section a better jump start, but I find it really hard to be optimistic when it comes to relationships. I've seen too many people hurt each other, use each other, get careless with each other, fuck and forget about each other. It's pretty disheartening and you'll just have to forgive me for not being in much of a Cupid kind of mood for this one.

We are a "me-first" generation. In a dog-eat-dog world, we have been trained to look out for ourselves, do what we want to do for ourselves, and always put ourselves first—no matter what the price, even if it means losing a meaningful relationship. Love isn't easy these days. With so many life options and opportunities, plus billions of people on this earth to choose from, love isn't as clear-cut as it used to be. Relationships are more complex and difficult than ever, and often they take a backseat to "bigger and more important" things. With life taking us everywhere and anywhere, I have to ask: When does a partner and a relationship take priority? When does love or the possibility of it come first? Why do we throw love and all of its potential away so easily? Why is it easier to drop a relationship than to work at one?

We're not making sacrifices for each other the way we used to. Instead, we're opting to get to know ourselves better and to fulfill our own needs. We're up for exploring more than one serious relationship and gaining insight about ourselves and who we want to be with. Many of us realize that taking the time to settle down can be beneficial for self-growth and, hopefully, steer us clear of loveless, long-term relationships. Hence, among the many challenges we face as young adults is that of finding and maintaining a monogamous, long-term relationship—allowing ourselves to completely fall in love.

Portia, a 25-year-old graduate student, does a good job addressing what I'm getting at:

> I always thought that if you were really in love with somebody—no matter what the situation was—that it would be enough. Make things bearable. But when you're in a relationship with somebody and you're both bringing things to the table—both people have to be happy with everything else that's going on in your life before you can expect that that relationship is going to thrive.

In such mobile, chaotic, fast-paced, modern times, it is hard to find somebody worthy of 100 percent of your time and affections, despite the abundance of people we have on this planet. With busy, demanding schedules, personal goals and desires, and unbelievable opportunities consuming us, we often leave our relationships and sexual encounters to chance. Furthermore, with many of us marrying later in life these days, we're encountering many more relationship experiences before determining what we want and whom we want. It can be a bit much at times. So let's look at some of the scenarios and issues we find ourselves dealing with.

Lust Versus Love

Only In August

You feel so right

In all of my searching and troubles and purpose

I'm finding you

You are my sedative

Your gaze—It relaxes me

Holds me tight

I am afraid of you, yet pray for you

To be with you forever, for life

Your touch mocks the power of my God

You are the breath I need

The life I breathe

But I gasp for air as your being, my spirit, our soul

PULL ME UNDER

Knowing that I won't resurface the same

I bargain with fate

Trusting I won't rise alone.

LUST

Lust is any intense attraction you have for another person in an erotic context. Simply put, lust is hot! Lust is infatuation! Lust is all about your sex drive! Maya, a 22-year-old with quite the sexual appetite, defines it pretty nicely: "Lust is purely physical, that animalistic attraction mainly characterized by wanting to rip someone's clothes off!"

I had a professor tell me once that lust lasts two years tops in a relationship. Every couple gets to a point where reality sets in and you realize that there's more to the person than just what you're physically craving. The individual isn't superhuman and there are things about the person that you actually *don't* find attractive. Veronica sets us straight on the role of lust in our relationships:

> Lust is based on attraction and chemistry. You idolize the person and tend not to look at their negative traits. You may feel really nervous around them because of the attraction. When you are together, you feel like you do not want to stop going further. You may lust after someone you don't like, in other regards. It's a roller-coaster ride of feeling, like you need that person with extreme highs and lows and maybe a bit of obsession—in the nonfatal attraction way.

LOVE

Love isn't so easy to define. Broadly speaking, there are two types of love: 1) **companionate love**, when you have a deep attachment and commitment to somebody else, and 2) **passionate love**, when you have an intense longing for union with the person that involves physical arousal. Yet while there's a distinction between these two types of love, a definition of love in general is still ambiguous, still hard to nail.

Research measuring love relationships has found that men hold a more romantic view of male–female relations than do women. Men also usually fall in love earlier in a relationship and cling longer to a dying love affair.

I know what love isn't. Love *isn't* lust. Love *isn't* romanticism, being wined and dined. It *isn't* a one-sided relationship of just fulfilling someone's needs or having your own needs met. It *isn't* about cooking him dinner every night, buying her expensive presents, or sleeping together. Love *isn't* having a dependency on another person or needing a partner to have a sense of self or to be worth something. Love *isn't* hurting a person intentionally, whether it's inflicting emotional or physical pain. Love *isn't* about desiring somebody because you love the stability a relationship provides. Love *isn't* getting stuck in the rut of a relationship's comfort and security, qualities of a partnership that are sometimes mistaken for stronger feelings long after the magic is gone. That's what love isn't. I'm sure that you have your own things to add.

Now, let me tell you what I think love is. Love *is* being able to be your own person, while still growing as a person and with your partner. Love *is* being willing to make room in your life for that person. Love *is* naturally making time for that person, making him or her a priority no matter how busy you are. Love *is* respecting that person in action and word and being thoughtful of that person. Love *is* accepting that person for who they are and everything about that person, both the good and the bad. Love *is* taking away the romance and comfort and still being able to care about the person. Love *is* being able to say anything to that person, to express yourself without fear of being judged. Love *is* feeling good about yourself, your partner, and your relationship. Love feels good.

BEING "IN LOVE"

Our idea of love evolves as we evolve. How we loved as teenagers is different from how we love as 20-something-year-olds, which is different from how we'll love when we're older. While we try to love to the best of our abilities as we grow up, if we're lucky to find somebody special enough to love, our capacity to love matures and becomes more meaningful with age and wisdom.

As we grow older, we also realize that there's a difference between loving someone and being "in love." You can love your parents, family, friends, boyfriend, girlfriend, pets, objects, and situations, all at different levels, but being "in love" is different. You feel different when you're "in love," as an old camp counselor friend of mine describes: "Being in love is when you can spend all week in the shop working. And then, when you are exhausted beyond repair, you still have all the energy provided by a power nap—just knowing you are going to see that someone."

Being in love takes all of that love stuff we just went over and goes one step further, as Maya describes: "When you're in love, lust and love are rolled into one package. It is respecting and admiring and liking and lusting after one other person all at once. It's the *crème de la crème* of emotions."

What I know of being in love is that it often doesn't make sense and it's never convenient. You can't plan when you're going to fall in love. It just happens.

Being in love with somebody means that you're willing to make sacrifices for that person. This person's needs and wants are as important, or even more important, than your own. You will go to the ends of the earth for that person, to be with that person.

Being in love means that you can't imagine your life without this person. You've lost yourself in this person, yet have never felt so found and grounded. Being in love is feeling satiated and complete. You don't need anything or anybody else because you're with this person, as Duncan, a 23-year-old sweetie who always makes people smile, has known:

> Being in love is when twenty-four hours a day, seven days a week...she's all you can think about. I know, I've been there. When you go out and the sight of beautiful women only makes you think more and more about that special someone. When you look at every girl in the room and point out all their flaws compared to the one you love. When you are on cloud nine when together! No matter what happens, as long as the two of you are okay...everything is wonderful. It's when all you want to do is hold that person for hours without words or movement.

Being in love is also about being able to let that person do what is best for himself or herself, even if that means that you're no longer going to be a part of that person's life. It's the hardest and worst thing about being in love, and giving the person up could be your greatest sacrifice. I hope, for most of you, your "in love" relationship will never have to go through something like this. I hope that it's forever.

Love is the most important ingredient to a great sex life, with good communication coming in second.

Cheating

Ewan, a 21-year-old student, explains:

I've had sex with nine girls in the three years that I've been dating my girlfriend. She thinks I'm an angel! (laughs hysterically). And I've hooked up with fifty others or more!... Why don't I just break up with her?... We're really tied into each other's lives and families. When I'm with her, I don't want to be with anybody else. But I get horny and we're doing the long-distance thing. And then I'm always drinking and going to Happies and parties here at school. Once you start cheating, it gets a lot easier. It's hard to go back and not do it anymore.

Cheating happens way more than any of us would care to admit. Almost 40 percent of women and 50 percent of men will cheat while in a monogamous relationship—not exactly the most uplifting figures on the state of our relationships. It's even more reason why all of us need to be practicing safer sex, why you need to be looking out for yourself. The prevalence of cheating is one of the reasons I'm fueled to write this sexual health–based book. I can't believe the number of people I know who have cheated on their very unsuspecting partners. Very frightening!

Since cheating is so common, I thought I'd ask some people about it, to find out why people are or aren't doing it. Here are some people's takes on cheating:

Portia:

I slept with my roommate's man even though I was dating her brother. I wasn't happy in my relationship with her brother and there was some sort of animal attraction to this other guy. Of course, I think that it was a terrible mistake. I feel eternally guilty. I wasn't happy and we weren't connected. On the other hand, it was great because I don't know if I would've gotten out of that relationship with her brother otherwise. It opened my eyes to what a relationship is all about and how there should be passion.

Miguel:

I've cheated, but not too much. It's only happened two times with two different girlfriends. I was drunk. In the one case, the girl was just absolutely gorgeous and I was in Puerto Rico—as if my girlfriend was going to find out! But with the other girlfriend, I did tell her. We were done.

Lacie, a 24-year-old graduate student:

Although I think I am the exception, I have never cheated on a boyfriend with whom I had a commitment. I would never sleep with two guys at the same time either, because telling my parents I was pregnant would be hard enough. If I had to tell them I didn't know which guy was the father, I would totally disgrace them. This might be my more dramatic side, but I always watch soap operas where they never seem to know who the father is. I don't ever want to put myself in a situation like that.

Duncan:

Never cheated. Can't. When I am with someone they are the only one I can be with. It is in my blood! I've had the opportunity, but couldn't do it. I'm a strict believer in do unto others as you would want done unto you!

Cheating is one of the reasons I get really discouraged about relationships. There's just no excuse for it. If you're in a relationship and find yourself cheating, it's an indication that something isn't right, that you're not as happy in your relationship as you could be. Plus, it puts your partner unknowingly at risk for a number of sexual-health threats. You're only doing your partner and yourself a favor by taking a "time-out" from your relationship to find out why you have this need to cheat. Perhaps, with some introspection, you'll be able to determine what kind of relationship you want to be in and with whom.

Threesomes

Though it may seem crude to actually say it, one way a few couples deal with temptations to cheat, plus fulfill each other's fantasies, is by having a threesome. **Threesomes** *(ménages à trois)* are one of those "dance with me, make me sweat" sexual escapades people talk, dream, or joke about, but in actuality not that many partake in.

Lots of people, like Bernard, a 26-year-old charmer, have thought about what it would be like to have a threesome and the impact it would have on a relationship:

> I've always wanted to try a threesome, but can't get past my dreams. I can't concentrate on more than one person. My girlfriend would be into it, willing to try it, but I'm even worried that we'll have sex with one and forget the other. I don't know if I could please two females at the same time. I can hardly rub my tummy and pat my stomach at the same time! Then my girlfriend would be willing to do it with two guys, but I won't do that. Double standard, I know, but I just can't do that.

Some people, like Petra and her partner, have been able to pull off successful threesomes, as she shares:

> Experimenting with a threesome (or moresome) can be a fun and exciting enhancer to a relationship. To involve someone else is to open a whole other world of sex play and all the feelings that go along with it. I remember how amazing it was to feel the softness of a woman's skin in a sexual way for the first time, to kiss her lips and touch her hair, and to watch her kiss and play with my partner. It was a turn-on to see her enjoying him and him pleasuring her. At the same time, though, it was also a real challenge!

> Open and honest communication was the key to making it work for us. Involving someone else brought up a lot of emotions that were unexpected, such as jealously, inadequacy, and doubt. Communicating openly with my partner, as well as the other person involved, was the only way to avoid bad feelings building up and assumptions being made. In the end, if you have a threesome, go into it SAFELY

and HONESTLY. Then, just relax and enjoy all the awesome new sensations!

Everybody has their own idea of what a threesome would be all about and what kind of threesome they'd consider participating in. If it's something you find yourself wanting to experiment with, make sure that this sexual endeavor is all about safer sex. Doubling the number of partners doubles the amount of risk involved for unintended pregnancy, STDs, and HIV. So make sure that you and your partners use protection!!!

Serial Monogamy

Serial monogamy is a premarital sexual pattern in which there's an intention of being faithful to a partner, but the relationship eventually ends and the person then moves on to another person. Forty percent of people are serial monogamists.

While I can appreciate the benefits that being a serial monogamist offers, like that of having a steady companion, I am skeptical about this relationship pattern. Serial monogamy indicates to me that, in most cases, a person has attachment or dependency issues. The person never has the time to develop the self and evaluate personal needs and wants. She or he never has the chance to grow in a way that only being single for a while can offer. Serial monogamy, in my opinion, also seems to make the feelings involved in each relationship not mean as much if a person can have one "meaningful" relationship after another. Maybe that's judgmental of me, but that's my take on it. Thinking every person has "'til death do us part" potential indicates to me that there are dependency, self-esteem, or other psychological issues going on.

The other concern I have about serial monogamists is that their relationships often involve unprotected sex; hence, sexual-health threats can spread quickly from relationship to relationship. I've had friends who are serial monogamists and in every monogamous relationship, sex eventually becomes unprotected, with at least one of the partners thinking that the relationship will be long-term and that they're so close with the partner that they don't need protection anymore. Sooner or later, having put themselves at risk for STDs and HIV, they break up and move on to the next partner, where the same thing happens. It's cyclical and risky for everyone involved, unless a couple incorporates protection for *at least* a minimum three-month incubation "window period" prior to HIV testing (see Chapter 7) to see whether or not they're good to go the unprotected route.

Meaningful Flings

Meaningful Flings are intense, romantic, instinctive connections with another person. They're more than a one-night stand, but less than an all-out relationship. Furthermore, they're not just about casual sexual activity. You and your fling partner totally bond.

Everybody has their own reasons for stumbling into a Meaningful Fling. Isabelle, a 23-year-old with the biggest heart in the world, gives her thoughts on why it happens:

> Meaningful Flings happen because your soul is not quite developed in that area, whether the fling involves sex or the simple gesture of a hug. Therefore, those flings entitle your soul to grow and experience something that needed to happen in order for your body, heart, mind, and soul to balance. And you learn more about yourself, what you want, what you do not want, and are a step closer to knowing who you are.

With Meaningful Flings, you can show your true colors—the real you. You can—without fear—share your hopes, your dreams, and your fears. You can be romantic and crazy, and say stuff like, "Can I keep you?" without worry that the partner is going to make a run for it or freak out. Maya loves Meaningful Flings:

> Everyone should have a Meaningful Fling at least once in their life. Really, they're the best learning experiences. They show you what you want to find in a lasting relationship—romance, heat, intensity, that loin-stirring "I-can't-wait-another-second" passion. But they also show you that attraction alone can't make it work, and how many other factors come into play as well... careers, families, geographic preferences... all the things you think sound secondary, but really define who we are. And besides, Meaningful Flings are a heck of a lot of fun!!

Meaningful Flings often involve having a great deal of distance from that person. There's some sort of physical barrier, like that you live in different time zones, which is very convenient, and yet you can still let your guard down. There's some safety in knowing it's all temporary, short-term. With Meaningful Flings, you enter a time warp of sorts, yet there's also usually a definite time limit. If any communication begins to occur on a regular basis, then you are headed for a relationship, and *relationship,* in a Meaningful Fling, is a dirty word.

Sometimes, but not always, one of the benefits of a Meaningful Fling is that you don't have to develop a committed relationship with the person if you don't want to, because when it boils right down to it—it's a fling—a fling that has meaning. When the romance ends, you don't have to blame yourself for its struggling or extinguished flame. You're not at fault or responsible. It's not because your fling thinks you're a dud, unattractive, annoying, or weird. You can point the finger at circumstance. That's where the blame lies because really, if you had met this person in a different context, things could've been heaven on earth. Yet because of circumstance, you'll never know and you can just leave your fling to sweet memory. You get to touch the sky and end things on a high note. (Make sure you don't come away from it with an STD, HIV, or pregnancy. Leaving the encounter to memory is certainly enough. Meaningful Flings should be safer-sex flings too.)

The One

My buddies and I debate about this pretty regularly: Is "The One" out there for you and, if so, how do you know? Some in our group say we're compatible with all sorts of people and simply prefer one of them, while others think that you'll meet somebody and you'll just know that this person is The One.

Many of us also think that every dating or steady relationship has an expiration date, usually after three to four years. It gets to a certain point where you either know that this is the person you want to spend the rest of your life with—that this person is The One—or you move on. We also think that a lot of being "undecided" actually stems from being unable or afraid to admit that a partner is *not* The One.

I'm one of those arguing that you know early on that a person is The One, that you just get this feeling. My cousin Anna knew her husband was The One because, "He's the one man who has ever been able to make me go weak in the knees!"

I also look at it as more of a soul-mate thing, and while you can be compatible with lots of different people, the soul-mate connection makes this person different, special—The One. I think we all have one person out there who complements us in every way, fulfills us, is in awe of us, loves us, and connects with us like no other. I hope everyone finds that soul mate in a lover.

The frustrating thing about finding The One is that you never know when it's going to happen. Or you have that cosmic connection with somebody you think is The One, but because of circumstance, the other party isn't willing to explore the possibility. Or you find somebody and think that this person has The One potential, but you really aren't sure, even as the two of you plan to tie the knot.

We often end up settling for somebody to marry who doesn't completely fulfill us or who at least doesn't fulfill us in the long run. It's probably part of the reason we have so many divorces these days. People aren't waiting around for The One.

Finding The One isn't necessarily finding the ideal. No single individual can make us happy in every single way, since we're all flawed. The One can't be selected or searched for either. Finding The One just happens.

No matter what kind of relationship you're in or desire, or whom it's with, I would hope that, more than anything, it's a healthy relationship. Among the components of a healthy relationship are the following:

* You and your partner can spend time alone with friends or family without involving the other.

* You both decide how you want to spend time with each other.

* You respect each other's values and opinions.

❋ You have open communication.

❋ You need each other because you love each other, not because you need a partner.

I want you to be treated as any decent human being should be treated in a relationship. I want you to be true to yourself. I want you to find what is real and to never settle until you do.

CHAPTER 6

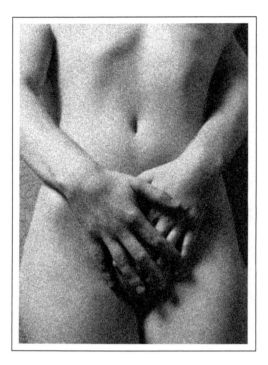

Who Me?
Get an STD?

What are STDs?

How do you get an STD? How can you avoid one?

What are the symptoms of STDs?

Believe it or not, it could happen to you—*you* could get an STD. I certainly hope that you will never contract a **sexually transmitted disease (STD)**, and you will really have no excuse after reading this book. Yet with so many people sexually active, and so many people sleeping with so many other people, and so many STDs out there—it could happen. Despite it being terribly unpleasant, I think it's really important to cover this area of sexuality.

I know what some of you are thinking: Who wants to think about STDs when they're thinking about sex? Sex is supposed to be animalistic! No-holds barred! Earth-shattering! Plus, just plain fun! However, because sex carries the risk of transmitting STDs via body-fluid exchange and sometimes skin-on-skin contact, we need to think about possible infection transmission. In addition to sex being erotic, we need to make sure that it's safe as well.

The information in this chapter is intended to remind you of why it is important and simply common sense to use protection when you're getting it on. The STDs described on the following pages will make you appreciate your healthy body, condoms, and other forms of protection that help to keep it healthy. Note that while HIV is an STD, it is not discussed in this chapter. Rather, Chapter 7 is entirely devoted to information on HIV. Chapters 8 and 9 address ways you can protect yourself from STDs and HIV.

Sadly, STDs are a fact of life that needs to be acknowledged and, unfortunately for a lot of people, needs to be dealt with too. Based on the current trends in STD statistics, even if you've never been infected, the chances that you'll eventually deal with an infected partner or an infection yourself are pretty good. So read the following information to find out what all of the concern is about, and keep it all in mind the next time you're debating whether or not to use a condom—thinking about whether it's worth it to protect yourself and your partner.

Sexually Transmitted Infections

Sexually transmitted infections (STIs) is the most up-to-date term for sexually transmitted diseases, formerly known as **venereal diseases (VDs)**. Since most of us still use the term "STDs," I'm going to stick with that abbreviation in this book.

There are more than twenty-five diseases that are spread through sexual contact and STDs are among the *most commonly spread* diseases in the United States. About one in every four adults in the United States has an STD. Every year, according to the Centers for Disease Control, there are about 15.3 million new cases of STDs, with two-thirds of these cases occurring in individuals under the age of 25.

WHY SHOULD YOU BE CONCERNED?

America is currently experiencing a rapid rise in the incidence of STDs, especially "classic" STDs like gonorrhea, syphilis, chlamydia, and genital herpes. By the age of 24, one out of every three sexually active young people will contract a sexually transmitted infection. These numbers are pretty alarming, because while some STDs can be cured if treated early, many of them can cause reproductive health and fertility problems if not given proper medical attention *promptly*. Furthermore, some STDs can even lead to severe and permanent damage, such as blindness, heart disease, cancers, or even death.

On top of all of those reasons to be concerned, STDs may be interrelated. You can have more than one STD at the same time or one STD may mask another that poses a more serious health problem. One STD may make it easier for another to flourish. This is especially concerning since there is an association between STDs and the human immunodeficiency virus (HIV), the virus that causes AIDS. A person who has had an STD is much more likely to have been put at risk for contracting HIV as well. The speculation is that this is because having an STD that creates ulcers or discharges increases your vulnerability to HIV infection.

A man with an STD may infect six out of ten women he has sex with, while a woman with an STD may infect one or two of her ten partners. A woman has a greater susceptibility to any STD because she has a larger genital surface area to be infected and because, during unprotected sex, the man's semen is deposited directly into her body.

CONCERNED YET?

Sure, all of that sounds like it sucks for *other* people. I'd hate to get an STD. What a pain. I'm soooo glad that STDs only happen to *other* people.

Wrong!! Don't for a minute think that contracting an STD could *never* happen to you—that it just happens to everybody else. Don't think that only promiscuous people get STDs. *Anybody* can contract an STD and that, I'm afraid, includes *you.* I can't stress all of this enough.

Mallory learned the hard way that she was vulnerable to STDs. She describes her reaction to the time she found herself at a health clinic with a nurse telling her that the sore on her vulva was probably genital herpes:

> I couldn't believe it. How could this happen to me? I'd always prac-ticed safe sex with Mac, but it was one of those situations where his penis slipped in. It wasn't sex because he pulled out right after it was in, but it still got into me unprotected.
>
> I didn't feel invulnerable to pregnancy or AIDS, but I definitely did to other diseases. I mean, this was Mac. He's clean-cut, nice, hot...has a youthfulness about him. He has boyish qualities. It never crossed my mind that I'd get something like this. Guess part of it is once you've scored a guy, you don't want anything to come between the two of you. You're on such a high that you're hooking up with him that other things seem more important than protecting yourself.

Like Mallory, a lot of people who have been diagnosed with an STD are often in shock because they always thought that STDs are things that happen to other people, like to "slutty," "dirty" people. This is certainly not the case. Anybody can have an STD. Anybody can be an STD carrier.

So a big reason why STDs are flourishing is that many people are under the false impression that they're invulnerable to STDs. I'll often hear a person who has dealt with an STD say, in retrospect, "I thought that I was safe because I was on the pill" or "We were monogamous...or at least I was...." Sadly, too many people find out too late that an STD doesn't care if you're on the pill or if you think you're in a monogamous relation-ship. An STD doesn't care who you are or how clean your record is either. STDs don't discriminate.

Who Gets STDs?

Anyone who has sex can get an STD—men, women, heterosexual, homosexual, young and old. Certain STDs can even get passed from a woman to her unborn infant, causing irreparable organ damage, blindness, or even death. No one is immune, even if you've already contracted an STD. *It takes only one time*—one sexual experience. So you need to be concerned about using protection *every time* you have sex for your own sake, your own health, and your life.

> One's number of sex partners is one of the most important risk factors in contracting an STD. People with ten lifetime sexual partners are estimated to be twenty times as likely to have contracted an STD than those with only one life partner. Those with five to ten life partners are nine times as likely to have acquired a bacterial infection, and five times as likely to have a viral infection, than a person with one life partner. Those with two to four life partners are about 2½ times as likely to have an STD as those with one life partner.

DO STDS POSE SPECIAL PROBLEMS FOR WOMEN?

Yes. Since some STDs have no signs or symptoms at all (are *asymptomatic*), it can be hard to diagnose them. Many STDs have the opportunity to do serious damage inside a woman's sex organs before they're even detected and treated. Such damage can lead to problems like ectopic (tubal) pregnancies, miscarriages, and infertility. Between 100,000 and 150,000 American women become infertile each year because of STD-related infections.

Women are more likely than men to become infected with at least one STD during their lifetime. Women are twice as likely as men to have genital warts, twice as likely to get chlamydia, and three times as likely to have genital herpes. Usually, a woman has no idea that she has acquired an STD until the infection has been active in her system for a long time.

> Men have a much lower risk of contracting an STD than women. Females face a 40 percent higher risk of getting a bacterial infection and a 30 percent higher risk of getting a viral infection.

How to Avoid STDs

Some ways to make sure you *don't* get an STD include

*   abstaining from sexual activity involving the exchange of any body fluids or genital skin-to-skin contact

*   practicing safer sex in a monogamous relationship—this is where **both** you and your partner can be 100 percent sure that you are and have been faithful to each other, have been tested for STDs and are uninfected, and can realistically expect and trust that the other will not cheat

*   not sharing needles or injection equipment of any kind, since some STDs are spread this way

What You Need to Know About STDs

In discussing the following STDs, I break them down into three major categories: bacterial infections, viral infections, and parasitic infections. Bacterial and parasitic infections are those that can be cured. If you ever get one of these, you can go to a doctor or clinic and they'll be able to hook you up with medication that will get rid of the bacteria or parasite.

Viral infections, on the other hand, are permanent. These are the infections that you will have for life. While their symptoms can be alleviated and temporarily treated, viral infections will always be with you and can plague you with an outbreak at any time.

For each STD described, it's a fairly quick read. This chapter is designed to be a reference more than anything, in case you ever need or want to read up on one of these diseases really quickly.

Bacterial Sexually Transmitted Diseases

GONORRHEA ("CLAP," "THE DRIP," "A DOSE")

What It Is

Gonorrhea is a bacterial STD. It is the most commonly reported infectious disease in the country—nearly one million cases are reported each year. It can occur in a man or woman's urethra, rectum, mouth and throat, reproductive organs, and even in the eyes. If left untreated, gonorrhea can cause arthritis, heart problems, dermatitis, and reproductive problems. Women with untreated gonorrheal infections can develop pelvic inflammatory disease (PID), which can lead to infertility, tubal pregnancy, and fetal wastage.

How It Is Transmitted

* vaginal or anal intercourse

* oral–genital contact

* from mother to baby during childbirth

* from infected fluids coming into contact with the eyes

Signs and Symptoms

Symptoms of a gonorrheal infection usually appear two to twenty-one days after infection.

GONORRHEA

In men	In women
creamy, yellowish, thick, puslike penile discharge (and thus stained clothing)	increased cloudy vaginal discharge
	burning urination
burning urination	lower abdominal discomfort
itching on or around penis	irregular bleeding
fever	painful urination
pelvic area pain	fever
	pelvic area pain
	painful intercourse
	Most women show no early symptoms!

How It Is Treated

Infected persons and their partners need to be treated with antibiotics. The spread of the infection can end within hours if treated effectively right away.

SYPHILIS ("SYPH," "POX," OR "BAD BLOOD)

What It Is

Syphilis is a bacterial STD, afflicting 40,000 people in the United States each year. It has three distinct stages associated with three sets of symptoms. If left untreated, syphilis will eventually attack the nervous and cardiovascular systems and cause death or permanent disability in its third stage. Syphilis increases a woman's risk of miscarriage and stillbirth, and leads to syphilis infection of the newborn.

How It Is Transmitted

* vaginal or anal intercourse

* oral–genital contact

* grinding (genital-to-genital or genital-to-anal contact)

* touching an infectious sore—a **"chancre"**

* from mother to baby during childbirth

Signs and Symptoms

The following signs have been grouped according to the stage during which they appear and are seen in both men and women:

SYPHILIS	
Primary Stage (1–12 weeks after exposure)	a hard, round, painless sore (chancre) on the penis, anus, mouth, tongue, lips, and even the fingertips, breast, or anywhere else you have had intimate sexual contact
Secondary Stage (1–6 months after original chancre)	(The chancre has disappeared at this point.) swollen lymph nodes skin rash, especially on palms and soles mouth sores headache soreness and aching of bones and joints

SYPHILIS (CONT'D.)	
Secondary Stage (1–6 months after original chancre)	hair loss
	flulike symptoms
	loss of appetite
	general malaise
Tertiary "Latent" Stage (1–5 years)	no visible signs

If syphilis is not treated well before the third stage, severe problems can develop, including heart disease, sores on the internal organs and eyes, ßand insanity. When left untreated, syphilis eventually attacks the brain and other organs, resulting in paralysis, senility, blindness, and/or heart damage.

How It Is Treated

Syphilis is treated with the administration of penicillin, doxycycline, tetracycline, or erythromycin.

CHLAMYDIA AND NONGONOCOCCAL URETHRITIS (NGU)

What It Is

Chlamydia is a bacterial STD that can take up residence in the genitals, anus, urinary tract, or throat. Experts estimate that it is the most common and fastest spreading STD—with approximately four million new cases in the United States each year. If left untreated, chlamydia may cause painful infections of the reproductive organs that can result in infertility in both sexes. Up to 80 percent of women and 10 percent of men with chlamydia have no symptoms and have no idea they're infected. Men with a chlamydia infection in the urethra are said to have **nongonococcal urethritis (NGU)**. If left untreated in a woman, chlamydia can cause **pelvic inflammatory disease (PID)** and lead to permanent damage and infertility.

How It Is Transmitted

* vaginal or anal intercourse

* oral–genital contact

* touching eyes after touching the vaginal fluid or semen of an infected partner

* from an infected mother to her newborn during childbirth

Signs and Symptoms

These symptoms normally appear seven to twenty-one days after sexual contact.

CHLAMYDIA/NGU	
In men	**In women**
slight, mucuslike penile discharge	mild, mucuslike vaginal discharge
burning or painful urination	frequent, painful urination
sore throat (if oral–genital contact)	lower abdominal pain
testicular pain	pelvic inflammation
Most men are asymptomatic!	nausea and fever
	irregular vaginal bleeding
	sore throat (if oral–genital contact)
	Most women are asymptomatic!

How It Is Treated

Infected persons and their partners need to be treated with antibiotics. It may take up to two weeks to clear up the infection. During that time, infected partners need to abstain from sexual activity.

VAGINOSIS

What It Is

Vaginosis is a general term that applies to any type of vaginal infection or inflammation of the vagina. The major types are **bacterial vaginosis (BV)**, **candidiasis (yeast infection, moniliasis, thrush)**, and **trichomoniasis ("trich")**. Though typically referred to as female health problems, men can also suffer from such infections or inflammations.

What Causes It

* **bacterial vaginosis** (BV)—*Gardnerella vaginalis* and other bacteria

* **candidiasis**—the yeastlike fungus *Candida albicans*

* **trichomoniasis**—the parasite *Trichomonas vaginalis*

Normally, a healthy vagina contains a balance of several kinds of bacteria. "Good" bacteria help keep the vagina slightly acidic in order to prevent harmful bacteria from growing too quickly. A healthy vagina produces a mucus-like discharge that may be slightly milky or clear, depending on the time of a woman's monthly menstrual cycle. Even this discharge has a slight odor.

Sometimes, the fungus count grows and causes problems such as vaginal itching, burning, pain during sex, and a heavy, curdy, white discharge. This indicates that the balance of "good" and "bad" bacteria in the vagina is upset and that the harmful bacteria are growing too quickly and causing infections. Things that can upset the balance of the vagina include

* lubricants

* vaginal sprays

* birth control devices

* birth control pills

* pregnancy

* tight pants

* severe obesity

* warm weather

* stress

* antibiotics

* douching

* damp underwear

* poor hygiene

* poor diet

* diabetes
* steroid medications

How Infection Occurs

* sexual contact (including oral sex)
* an allergic reaction
* a change in vaginal flora that allows an overgrowth of infectious organisms
* yeast infections may be passed from one woman to another through the sharing of damp washcloths or towels

Signs and Symptoms

Symptoms include irritation and itching of the genitals, soreness and swelling of vaginal and nearby tissues, mild pain during urination, and discomfort during sexual intercourse. If transmitted orally, these infections may produce a yellowish, whitish, or greenish film on the tongue. Up to 50 percent of women are asymptomatic.

VAGINOSIS (GARDNERELLA VAGINALIS)

In men (general bacterial infection)	In women For yeast infections
irritation or itching of genitals	thin, foul-smelling vaginal discharge, which may be white and cottage cheeselike in appearance, or foamy and yellowish
tingly feeling in penis	
burning sensations during urination	
reddening or inflammation of foreskin and glans of the penis	smell of baking bread
thin, watery discharge	irritation of vulva
painful intercourse	**For trichomoniasis**
Bacterial infections are often asymptomatic!	heavy yellow-green or gray discharge
	bad smell
	For BV
	white or gray, watery or foamy discharge
	strong fishy smell, especially after sex
	Trich and BV are often asymptomatic!

How It Is Treated

✳ Bacterial vaginosis and trichomoniasis are treated through oral administration of the drug metronidazole (Flagyl) or clindamycin.

✳ Candidiasis is treated with vaginal creams, suppositories, or tablets containing the drugs miconazole, clotrimazole, or terconazole; area is kept dry.

Note: Some of these medications weaken latex condoms and diaphragms.

Women can also prevent recurrences by wearing cotton underwear; avoiding pantyhose, tight jeans, wet bathing suits, feminine hygiene products, and douching; and wiping from front to back after using the toilet. Keeping the area dry will help speed up the cure. Also, using cold compresses or soaking in a tub can relieve the itching. A woman should use the treatment even if she is having her period.

Note: If there's a chance that you contracted any of these vaginal infections from sexual contact, make sure that your partner has been treated as well so you don't have a recurrence!

As many as 80 percent of women are not able to recognize the symptoms of bacterial vaginosis, the most common of the vaginal infections, and often mistake it for a yeast infection. Thus, many of them try to self-treat the vaginal infection with an over-the-counter, antifungal medication, which is ineffective against BV.

PELVIC INFLAMMATORY DISEASE (PID)

What It Is

PID is a serious bacterial infection of the uterus that spreads from the vagina or cervix to damage the fallopian tubes. It strikes more than a million women in the United States every year. Up to one in seven women has PID at least once before age 35. Seventy-five percent of women afflicted with PID are under the age of 25.

What Causes It

Most often, gonorrhea or chlamydia infections assist in the development of PID because they often result in an infection of the fallopian tubes and ovaries. Other bacteria that are normally found in the genital tracts and body have also been known to cause infection. IUDs, douching, recent pelvic surgery, abortion, miscarriage, or having given birth also increase a woman's risk of PID.

How It Is Transmitted

* penile–vaginal intercourse

Signs and Symptoms

The following symptoms can appear anywhere from several weeks to several months after infection if the STD has not been treated:

* noncramping, steady pain in the pelvis or lower abdomen
* pain during intercourse
* fever
* discharge of pus
* irregular menstrual bleeding
* painful menstruation
* pain or difficulty in urination
* pain in the upper abdomen or lower back

Note: PID is sometimes asymptomatic.

How It Is Treated

Antibiotics are used. If left untreated, PID can lead to chronic pain, infertility, and other severe, even life-threatening, consequences.

Note: It is possible to transmit STDs via unclean sex toys.

GENITAL HERPES

What It Is

Genital herpes is a viral infection—caused by related strains of the herpes simplex virus—that 500,000 Americans contract every year. Since an estimated 40 million Americans have herpes, about one in five people over the age of 12 are carriers of this virus (a carrier is someone who has a sickness but does not show any symptoms). About two out of three people with herpes do not know that they are infected and potentially contagious.

What Causes It

Genital herpes is caused by the herpes simplex virus-type 2 (HSV-2). Infection can also occur during oral sex, due to one's partner having oral herpes—the herpes simplex virus-type 1 (HSV-1), a condition 50 to 80 percent of American adults carry.

The virus lives in the nerve cells at the bottom of the spine and "creeps" to the surface every now and then to cause the characteristic blisters and sores. Recurrence may be triggered by any number of things, including fatigue, menstruation, sunburn, and irritation. Usually, outbreaks are milder and shorter in duration in men. There can be a crossover between HSV-1 and HSV-2 due to oral sex, meaning that someone who has oral herpes can give you genital herpes when "going down" on you. HSV-2 is the harder to handle and more painful of the two viruses.

How It Is Transmitted

* anal or vaginal sex with an infected partner, usually when the individual has an active outbreak of the disease

* oral sex—an individual with a cold sore on the mouth or carrying the oral herpes (HSV-1 strain) can give his or her partner genital herpes

* grinding (genital-to-genital or genital-to-anal contact)

* genital contact with objects, such as toilet seats, used by an infected person may—but probably infrequently—transmit herpes viruses

* oral herpes (HSV-1) may also be transmitted by using the same cup, by kissing, or even by sharing a moist towel used by an infected person

* from an infected mother to her baby, *in utero* or during birth

Herpes is most contagious during outbreaks and for two weeks afterwards, so you should abstain from sex when symptoms are present. Less commonly, herpes is also transmittable when symptoms are not present.

Signs and Symptoms

People often think that if you have herpes, then you always have an outbreak. In reality, the body's immune system does a good job handling the infection. Symptoms generally occur three weeks to nine months after an individual contracts the virus. Yet many people with the herpes virus never develop sores. The first symptom of genital herpes, the "prodromal phase," is a tingling or itching sensation in the genital area. This phase *may be* followed by sores. On average, an individual with herpes has four recurrences per year. Attacks become less severe and less frequent over time.

HERPES

In men	In women
Painful, reddish bumps, sores or lesions which may appear on the penis, thighs or buttocks, and/or in or around the anus	Painful, reddish bumps, sores, or lesions which may appear on or in the vagina and/or anus, thighs, buttocks, or cervix
Lesions may be tender and itchy	Lesions may be tender and itchy
Bumps become blisters or sores that fill with pus and break	Bumps become blisters or sores that fill with pus and break
Burning urination or problems urinating	Burning urination or problems urinating
Fever	Fever
Headache	Headache
Aches and pains	Aches and pains
Swollen glands	Swollen glands
Pain in the legs, buttocks, or genital area prior to an outbreak	Pain in the legs, buttocks, or genital area prior to an outbreak
Feeling of pressure in the abdomen	Feeling of pressure in the abdomen
With oral herpes, the appearance of cold sores, "fever blisters," on the lips, inside of the mouth, on the tongue, or in the throat	Vaginal discharge
	With oral herpes, the appearance of cold sores, "fever blisters," on the lips, inside of the mouth, on the tongue, or in the throat

How It Is Treated

Herpes is incurable and may recur. Some sufferers have many recurrences, while others have few. With time, the attacks usually become less severe. An antiviral drug, acyclovir, marketed as Zovirax in ointment or capsule form, while not a cure, promotes healing and relief of herpetic sores, even shortening the duration of the outbreak. When Zovirax is given in oral form and taken daily, it may reduce the frequency of recurrence. Two new drugs—valacyclovir (Valtrex) and famciclovir (Famvir)—can also provide the same relief, but with lower doses because they are better absorbed by the body. Without treatment, the sores form scabs and heal in a few days to three weeks without leaving scars.

You can alleviate itching with compresses made of black tea or by taking baking soda baths. You should keep the area clean and dry in order to help the sores heal faster. Wear cotton underwear.

Remember that you can spread the virus to other parts of your own body, like your eyes, with your hands. So wash your hands well after touching sores. For oral herpes, nonprescription lip balms and cold-sore medications can be used to ease the outbreak.

In general, the best defense against herpes is a strong immune system. By keeping yourself healthy by getting enough sleep and eating a balanced diet that includes supplements of vitamin C, zinc, and immune system-boosting herbs like echinacea, you can often keep the virus at bay.

Note: The following three diseases are not exclusively sexually transmitted.

HUMAN PAPILLOMA VIRUS (HPV; "GENITAL WARTS," "VENEREAL WARTS")

What It Is

HPV is the name of a family of viruses that includes more than twenty different strains, about a third of which cause genital problems that affect men and women. About twenty million Americans have some strain of HPV, with 5.5 million Americans acquiring the STD every year. Genital warts, or condylomas, are one kind of lesion caused by HPV and are associated with cervical cancer in women, with HPV DNA having been found in up to 93 percent of women with cervical cancer. Hence, HPV leads to approximately 5,000 deaths every year in the United States.

HPV warts may also appear on one's hands and face. Sometimes HPV infection causes no warts and many people with genital HPV do not know they have it.

How It Is Transmitted

* skin-to-skin contact during vaginal, anal, or oral sex with an infected partner

* direct skin contact—such as grinding—with external genital warts, without vaginal or anal penetration

* contact with infected towels or clothing

* from an infected mother to her baby during childbirth

Even a condom can't entirely protect an individual from HPV because a condom does not cover the vulva, anus, scrotum, and penis—places where you could have direct contact with infected skin. Abstinence is the only way to protect yourself from the sexual transmission of HPV.

Signs and Symptoms

Genital warts generally appear two to three months after infection or they may never appear. Even if an individual never sees any warts, she or he can still be contagious.

HPV	
In men	**In women**
Flesh-colored and painless warts or bumps on the penis, scrotum, groin, thighs, and/or in and around the anus in varying sizes and shapes that may resemble common plantar warts	Flesh-colored and painless warts or bumps on the vulva, thighs, in or around the vagina or anus, and/or on the cervix, that may resemble common plantar warts
Warts may be raised or flat, single or multiple, small or large	Warts may be raised or flat, single or multiple, small or large
Some cluster together forming a cauliflower-like shape	Some cluster together forming a cauliflower-like shape
Itching, pain, or bleeding (rare)	Itching, pain, or bleeding (rare)
May be asymptomatic!	*May be asymptomatic!*

Invisible HPV

Sometimes, HPV causes very subtle changes in the skin that can't be seen with the naked eye. These "microscopic warts" can be found only with the help of special instruments. Other times, HPV can live in the skin without causing any warts at all. When this is the case, health-care providers call the HPV infection "clinically inapparent" or "subclinical."

How It Is Treated

No cure exists. Even with treatments that attempt to get rid of HPV by destroying infected cells, the virus can lie dormant in the cells and return months or even years later. Between 10 to 30 percent of warts regress (go away) spontaneously, though physicians cannot predict those that will regress. Genital warts are generally removed by a doctor, but the underlying HPV infection remains in the body indefinitely. Removal may include the following treatments:

* **cryotherapy** (cold cautery)—freezing off the wart with liquid nitrogen

* **podofilox** and **podophyllin**—anti-wart, chemical compounds applied to the surface of the wart

* **trichloracetic acid** (TCA)—chemical applied to surface of wart by physician

* **electrocautery**—an electrosurgery that destroys the infected tissue with an electric current by shaving it with a tiny loop or burning it away

* **laser therapy**—an intense beam of light is used to destroy the warts

* **excisional biopsy**—the warts are cut away

* **antiviral drug interferon**—a drug is injected into the warts two to three times weekly for about eight weeks (very expensive and has a high incidence of unpleasant side effects)

Do not attempt to remove the warts on your own!!! You could spread the virus!

VIRAL HEPATITIS—HEPATITIS B (HBV)

What It Is

Viral hepatitis is a liver disease, caused by related strains of hepatitis viruses, that infects more than 200,000 Americans every year. HBV is one of these strains. About 6,000 people die each year from hepatitis.

How It Is Transmitted

* sexual contact involving blood, vaginal fluids, or semen with an infected partner (often involving the anus)

* transfusion of contaminated blood

* blood from cuts or open sores and sharp objects contaminated with infected blood (hypodermic needles, toothbrushes, razors)

* contact with infected fecal matter

Signs and Symptoms

Referred to as a "silent infection," HBV infects many people who have no symptoms at all. Many adults don't develop symptoms at first, but about 50 percent experience some symptoms after an incubation period of 40 to 140 days. Whether or not one has symptoms, a person with HBV can pass the virus on to other people.

In both men and women, symptoms include the following:

* appetite loss

* nausea

* diarrhea

* vomiting

* fatigue

* abdominal pain

* fever and chills

* headache

* joint or muscle aches

* dark urine

* light stools

* anorexia

* a yellowish (jaundiced) tinge to the skin and eyes

* may be asymptomatic!

For individuals who are long-term carriers, ongoing liver damage may lead to **cirrhosis** (scarring of the liver), liver failure, or liver cancer. Severe cases of hepatitis can result in bleeding, coma, or death.

How It Is Treated

No cure exists, but most people who contract HBV—90 percent of them—recover within six months and then become immune to it. However, a small percentage of them cannot clear the virus from their body and become long-term (chronic) carriers.

There is one antiviral medication—interferon—that helps to normalize liver enzymes, and thus reduces the possibility of liver damage. However, less than 50 percent of people with chronic HBV are able to take interferon and only about a third of them experience significant long-term benefits from it. Steroids are used as treatment in severe cases. A vaccine to prevent infection is available.

VIRAL HEPATITIS—HEPATITIS C (HCV)

What It Is

This STD is a viral infection that causes inflammation of the liver. If it becomes chronic, it can ultimately destroy the liver. Up to 80 percent of cases develop into the chronic stage. Four million Americans, mostly between the ages of 20 and 39, and more males than females, are infected with HCV.

How It Is Transmitted

* sharing needles (and possibly, drug-snorting equipment)

* unprotected anal or vaginal sex

* tattooing and body piercing with improperly sterilized equipment

* sharing devices that can harbor contaminated blood (razors, nail clippers, toothbrushes)

* acupuncture (via improperly sterilized equipment)

Signs and Symptoms

Many people with HCV do not experience any symptoms, often for ten to thirty years. As a result, 90 percent of HCV carriers don't even know they're infected. The incubation period for hepatitis C is two weeks to six months, but most commonly six to nine weeks. Symptoms may include the following:

* headaches
* depression
* fatigue
* aches and pains

How It Is Treated

There is no cure for HCV. Injections of the drug interferon, or interferon combined with ribavirin, are the only treatments, and they unfortunately have side effects like hair thinning, a decrease in white blood cell count, and flulike symptoms. A bit of good news, however, is that about 15 percent of people infected with HCV will clear the virus from their bodies naturally.

Parasitic Sexually Transmitted Infections

PEDICULOSIS PUBIS ("CRABS," "COOTIES," "PUBIC LICE")

What It Is

Extremely contagious, tiny parasites that breed in the pubic hair and cause intense itching. The pubic louse attaches itself to the skin around the genitals and lays eggs ("nits") on the pubic hair shafts. A louse can live for up to thirty days in the pubic hair.

How It Is Transmitted

* sexual contact
* contact with infested bedding, clothes, towels, or toilet seats

Signs and Symptoms

It's marked by intense, persistent itching in the genital area and other hairy regions to which lice become attached, e.g., chest, scalp, eyebrows, or underarms. One may also see moving lice in the pubic hair and eggs attached to hair shafts. Other symptoms include mild fever, swollen lymph glands, and muscle aches.

How It Is Treated

Treatments include Lindane solution (Kwell), a prescription shampoo, or other nonprescription medications containing pyrethrins or piperonyl butoxide (brand names: RID, Triple X). Try not to scratch while using this medication! Sexual partners should be treated as well. In addition, clothes and bedding should be washed, since nits can live for almost one week unattached to a human.

SCABIES

What It Is

Scabies is a contagious skin disease in which a parasitic mite burrows itself under the skin to deposit eggs.

How It Is Transmitted

  * sexual contact

  * contact with infested bedding, towels, or clothing

Signs and Symptoms

Scabies results in intense itching in the genital area, appearance of reddish burrows in skin, and/or a rash.

How It Is Treated

To treat scabies, use Lindane solution (Kwell), and do a thorough cleaning of your clothes, linens, etc.

Is It Time to Get Tested?

So those bumps on your vulva might be a sign of genital warts. Or that discharge coming out of your penis doesn't look too healthy. Or maybe you're feeling perfectly healthy, but are wondering if you could've gotten something from even that *one* time you had unprotected sex. Although going to a doctor or clinic may not be the most enjoyable of excursions, it might be a good idea to get tested.

Even the experience of thinking that you might have an STD is overwhelming and scary. Jack, a 25-year-old medical student and health advocate whose confessed desire was to sleep his way to Capitol Hill, describes his reaction and concerns to a scare that he might have had an STD:

> Thinking about the chance that I could have pubic lice and going to the doctor's made me feel anxious. I felt that talking about any sexual concerns with my doctor could open up a whole can of worms. So the whole time I was at the clinic, I was wondering "What do I tell him? What am I going to disclose about my behavior? How are others judging me because of this?" As a health-care practitioner myself, I learn about all of the aspects about the body—all the ins and outs and what can happen. But I still always think that it'll be the patients with problems. It's all about them. Then when it's you, you feel fear, embarrassment, shame, anxiety....

> I was relieved to find out that I didn't have pubic lice, but instead had an abscess. At the same time, I still didn't feel good because the doctor didn't normalize it when he told me that I had an abscess. He didn't normalize my earlier fears that it might've been public lice. He didn't tell me the number of people it happens to. So I was there wondering "Am I the only person that's come to talk to you in the last five years about this?! Am I the only one?! Tell me it'll be okay. Tell me I'm not the only one! Tell me someone else had told you that before!"

If you think that you may have an STD or do have one, it is nothing to be embarrassed about. The smart thing to do is to go for a checkup. Even if you aren't showing any symptoms but are wondering if you have an STD that's asymptomatic, see a doctor as soon as possible, just for your peace of mind. Furthermore, make sure to tell the physician about *all* of your symptoms. Don't be afraid to ask questions. Doctors are supposed to deal with sexual health ailments; it's part of their job. If you do not feel comfortable going to your doctor, find a doctor with whom you are more at ease.

Dealing with an STD

Let's say you find out that you do, after all, have an STD. The first reaction people normally have when diagnosed with an STD is to feel overwhelmed. You may be shocked, angry, and/or scared. Being diagnosed with an STD, especially a viral one, can be emotionally and psychologically damaging. You may feel that you are "damaged goods." You may think that your sex life is over, that you'll never be able to have sex again, that no one will ever want to come near you. You may feel like you're going to be paying the price for a long time, if not forever.

It's not unusual for a person with an STD to experience feelings of shame and a negative body image. A person usually feels used-up and unclean. Most people who have been diagnosed with a viral STD experience depression and fear rejection by future partners.

Fortunately, these feelings pass. You eventually learn to adjust to viral infections and rebuild your self-image with time. People afflicted with an STD often find the following three keys to be most helpful in their quest to reestablish ownership of their body and sexual health:

I. EDUCATE YOURSELF

Education is the first step to restoring the blow your self-esteem has suffered. Knowledge is power! By gathering information about the infection and how it affects your body, you can gather strength. So get as much information as you can about ways of medically and psychologically coping with the disease. Learning the best ways to cope with the infection can help you regain a sense of control over your body. Furthermore, myths surrounding STDs can play a part in feelings of shame and you can combat these fallacies by going on a fact-finding mission.

II. KNOW YOUR BODY

Get to know your body. Become more genital-friendly. Take the time to observe your genitals with a handheld mirror when you have an outbreak *and* when your genitals are in a healthy state. Observe the timing of your outbreaks so that you know what your triggers are, e.g., you have an outbreak when you're under enormous amounts of stress, or when you consume great amounts of caffeine. By having a better sense about the timing of your outbreaks, you will have a greater sense of control over your infection and an acceptance of your body's changes. Be sure to research your STD so that you're more informed about its triggers.

III. BE PATIENT

Be patient with yourself. With the passage of time, the shock will wear off. Find somebody to talk to, maybe even a therapist. Take the time to adjust to your new body image and the new beliefs about yourself as a person. Also, learn to accept rejection from a potential partner without thinking that you're a terrible person.

THE BENEFITS OF TELLING

Every time a person who is infected with an STD starts a new sexual relationship, he or she is faced with the dilemma of whether or not to tell a partner about the disease and risk rejection, loss of confidentiality about being infected, humiliation, and other adverse effects. Despite such understandable concerns, studies have found that people with a viral infection usually choose to disclose that they carry an STD. They are focused on the rights of the partner and the obligations necessary to maintain a good relationship.

Telling a partner nurtures the feelings necessary for a successful intimate relationship: truthfulness, a willingness to be open, and sharing. As a result, some partners of infected individuals find the fact that their partner can be so open and forthright about something so difficult to be positive enough that it destigmatizes the fact that they have an STD.

Many people with an STD become more cautious in their sexual relationships, more direct with their partners. Having had an STD themselves, they don't want to put their partner through the same experiences they've had and they want to protect their partner to the best of their ability. Such lines of communication are beneficial to the relationship in that they can open up a conversation of sexual history and STDs. Partners can become closer, knowing more about each other and their sexual experiences, plus they can work together to make sure that they protect themselves in the future.

If you choose to tell, make sure you have the facts about your STD down. You'll need these to correct myths or calm fears your partner may have about the disease. Try not to be anxious about your news. Sounding overly stressed or panicky can make the condition seem worse than it really is. Try to be calm and confident. Lastly, don't blurt out such information in the heat of passion. Such a conversation should take place in an emotionally neutral environment.

SO YOUR PARTNER HAS AN STD

It's difficult to talk about sex. It's even more difficult to talk about STDs. When your partner is diagnosed with a chronic STD, your relationship can be thrown into utter turmoil. Things might get ugly, perhaps because your partner has been cheating. Or perhaps your lover wasn't open about having an STD when things first became really intimate. Or perhaps a partner just didn't know that he/she was a carrier of an STD, a remnant of a long-past relationship that is just now starting to cause trouble.

No matter what the circumstances are why a partner has an STD, if you plan to stay together, you have a lot of issues to deal with. A viral sexually transmitted infection is forever. First you need to find common ground to comfortably talk about the subject. Then you need to figure out how you will protect yourselves from now on, and even when you will have sex if faced with a viral STD that may act up on occasion.

Relationships involving STDs can be dealt with. This kind of relationship needs a lot of trust, care, communication, and *lots* of protection. People who truly care about each other and their health are willing and able to cope with STDs adequately and overcome the burdens an infection can place on a relationship.

Whether or not you are infected with an STD, you do have control over the impact an STD can have on your life. You have the power to prevent getting and/or transmitting an STD. You have the ability and know-how to protect yourself and your partner, especially after reading this book. You have a choice about your sexual health.

RESOURCES

For more information on STDs, call or visit the following:

ASHA—American Social Health Association—a nonprofit organization offering STD information: www.ashastd.org

Centers for Disease Control—National STD Hotline: (800) 227-8922

Herpes Advice Center: (888) ADVICE8 (238-4238)

Herpes & HPV Hotline: (800) 230-6039

HPV Hotline: (877) HPV-5868 (478-5868) (toll free), 2:00–7:00 P.M. EST

For information on STDs: www.thebody.com

To learn to identify STDs by sight: http://thebody.com/sowadsky/symptoms/symptoms.html

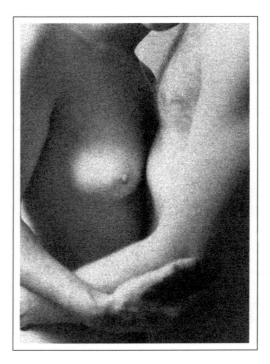

CHAPTER 7

The Lowdown
on
HIV/AIDS

What is AIDS? What is HIV?

How do you become infected with HIV?

How can you protect yourself from HIV?

What can you do with your partner and still not have
to worry about HIV?

Feeling lucky? Ever ask yourself that, as you're twiddling a condom between your fingers, making that split-second decision about whether or not to use it—whether or not to put it on? How were the cards dealt this time? What are you willing to bet? Just how lucky do you feel?

Consider yourself lucky. Lucky you have that protection available. Lucky you have that choice. Lucky you're going to know how to use that protection and make it amazing by the end of this book. Lucky you have the information you need to protect yourself and your partner. Lucky you get to decide your own fate.

I hope that for most of you the information in this chapter is a review of material you are already familiar with. Considering the current state of sex education in this country, however, I thought that it would be a good idea to make sure that all of this information is included. In dealing with our sex lives, we can never be reminded enough of our vulnerability to HIV and how we can protect ourselves from infection.

What Is AIDS?

The **acquired immunodeficiency syndrome (AIDS)** is a viral syndrome that attacks and damages the body's nervous systems and strips the immune system of its ability to defend itself against life-threatening diseases. It is the final and most advanced stage of a disease caused by the **human immunodeficiency virus (HIV).**

Once infected with HIV, a person has this virus for life. It is a virus that weakens, and causes an eventual collapse of, the body's ability to fight off illness. A person with AIDS is vulnerable to other diseases, even ones that the body would normally be able to fight off, like *Pneumocystis carinii,* a type of pneumonia. Serious infections, pneumonia, and cancers (even rare types, like the cancer Kaposi's sarcoma) are able to invade an AIDS-ridden body and eventually cause death.

AIDS stands for the following:

A—Acquired—Implies that the disease is not genetic or inherited

I——Immuno—Refers to the immune system that protects the body against disease

D——Deficiency—Means that the body's immune system is compromised, leading to an increased vulnerability to illnesses

S—Syndrome—Describes a set of symptoms that occur together, separately or serially (one after the other)

What Is HIV?

HIV breaks down into the following:

H——Human—A species-specific virus; humans transmit the virus to other humans

I—Immunodeficiency—Attacks the immune system

V—Virus—Caused by a type of antigen (not a bacteria or parasite)

HIV is a blood-borne retrovirus, meaning that it reverses the normal flow of genetic information within a host cell—a cell it has invaded—in order to reproduce itself. When somebody has HIV, they are said to be HIV positive (HIV+). It is estimated that 900,000 Americans are living with HIV, with at least 40,000 people becoming newly infected every year.

The United States of AIDS

The most current statistics released by the Centers for Disease Control and Prevention (CDC) in December 2000 indicate that there are over 450,000 cases of HIV/AIDS in the United States. More than 20 percent of the people who have AIDS are in their 20s, your peers. Young people under the age of 25 make up half of all new HIV infections in the United States, with the majority of them being infected sexually. AIDS is the fifth leading cause of death among people between the ages of 25 and 44.

What this boils down to is that most people—regardless of their sexual orientation—are becoming infected with HIV as teenagers and young adults. College students are a population that is at a greater-than-average risk of contracting HIV, with one in every five hundred college students testing positive for HIV. It is estimated that at each of the largest universities in the United States, at least seventy students may be infected with the virus.

About one in three people infected with HIV do not even know that they are infected!

It's important to know the information in this chapter. The more we know about this deadly virus, how it is and isn't transmitted, the better we can become at protecting ourselves and the people we care about. Knowing this information, applying it to our sexual behaviors, and practicing safer sex is one way we can combat this disease, and while we can't necessarily get rid off it completely, we can at least drive down the rates of infection, which are all too high everywhere on this planet.

How Does AIDS Affect the Immune System?

The body's immune system includes two types of white blood cells, one of which is the "helper" T-cells, or T4 cells. These cells assist in fighting disease by identifying foreign antigens and directing the body's immune system response against infection. When a person is infected with HIV, the virus binds itself to the surface of a helper T-cell and enters it, where it may lie dormant for years without causing any symptoms.

Eventually, the virus causes the T4 cell to lose its normal function and directs it to genetically produce more viral replicas of HIV before the T4 cell dies. These viruses then exit the T4 cell to attack other T4 cells. As more and more virus-impregnated T4 cells die, the victim is left with an inadequate immune system and thus cannot fight off other illnesses. AIDS is diagnosed when the T4 cell-count drops to less than 200/mL of blood (T4 counts from 800 to 1200 mL are considered healthy in adults).

How Is HIV Transmitted?

SEXUAL CONTACT

Heads up! This is what I consider to be the most important part of this chapter, the part that's going to help you know what behaviors put you at risk for contracting HIV. HIV is transmitted *sexually* via the following:

* vaginal–penile intercourse

* anal intercourse

* oral–genital contact

With these forms of transmission, the virus can get into the blood-stream through tiny tears in the lining of the vagina, rectum, or mouth. People who have sex with men are more likely to be infected by an HIV+ lover than are people who have sex with women—that is, an HIV+ man will infect his partner more often than will an HIV+ woman. The transmission of HIV from asymptomatic (without symptoms) HIV+ men is five times more likely than transmission of the virus from asymptomatic HIV+ women. This is because men deposit their semen directly into the vagina, the anus, or the mouth, and because every time intercourse takes place, the vaginal and/or anal lining has microscopic tearing that makes a person more susceptible to HIV.

> The risk of transmission from an HIV-positive woman is increased while she has her period. This is because there are more viral particles in the vagina during menstruation.

OTHER WAYS HIV IS TRANSMITTED

* blood transfusion with contaminated blood or plasma supplies

* from an infected mother to her fetus in utero or to her newborn during delivery

* sharing of contaminated hypodermic needles

* sharing unclean sex toys with an infected partner

> When needles are used to inject drugs, some blood is left behind in the needle tip or the syringe. The next person who uses the needle injects this blood into his/her system.

TRANSMISSION EQUATION

I apologize if this chapter feels text-bookish. There's no other way to get such vital information across. You might be understandably bummed out about this information right now—this is stressful stuff we're going over.

I promise that from here on out, I'm not going to be too technical with this information. I've thrown a lot of bodily fluids and behaviors your way, and it can be a lot to keep track of and recall. Really quickly, though: If there's one thing that I want you to know about HIV transmission, it's the formula below. This equation can help you to determine if what you're doing, or going to do, puts you at risk for contracting HIV. If you remember this equation and act on it by protecting yourself in practicing safer sex, then you should be able to rest easy about HIV/AIDS.

(The following fluids are listed in their amount of HIV concentration from highest to lowest.)

Blood		Mucous membrane		
Semen	+	OR	=	Potential risk of transmission
Vaginal fluids		Broken skin		
Breast milk				

Your Mucous Membranes

* eyes

* nose

* mouth

* tip of penis

* vaginal lining

* anal lining

Broken Skin

* cut

* rash

* open sores

Even pre-ejaculate fluid can contain HIV, and thus any sexual activity involving pre-cum can put you at risk for contracting the virus.

What Are You to Do?

Since there's a lot of misinformation out there as to how you can and can't get HIV, I want to go over what is and isn't safe to do.

HOW HIV IS <u>NOT</u> TRANSMITTED

* casual, everyday contact
* shaking hands
* through tears, sweat, saliva, urine, feces, or vomit
* hugging, kissing
* coughing, sneezing
* giving blood
* using swimming pools, water fountains, toilet seats
* sharing bed linens
* using telephones
* touching door knobs
* via mosquitoes, other insects, and animals

Now we know what we don't have to worry about. So based on all of that, the following sexual behaviors have been categorized by most sex and health educators as being high, low, or no risk for transmitting HIV.

HIGH-RISK SEXUAL BEHAVIORS

* unprotected penile–vaginal intercourse
* unprotected anal intercourse
* oral sex on a man without a condom (with or without swallowing the ejaculate)
* oral sex on a woman without a barrier during her time of menses

LOW-RISK SEXUAL BEHAVIORS

* penile–vaginal intercourse **with a latex condom**

* anal intercourse *with a latex condom*

* oral sex on a woman with a barrier (riskier, though not high risk if no barrier is used)

* oral sex on a man with a condom

* rimming (oral–anal contact)

* grinding (direct genital-to-genital or genital-to-anal contact)

NO-RISK SEXUAL BEHAVIORS

* massaging

* hugging

* cuddling and touching

* sexually stimulating another person using your hand (as long as you don't have any open sores on your hand)

* fantasizing

* kissing

* having phone sex

* masturbating, mutual masturbation, or watching someone else masturbate

* using sex toys that have been cleaned before use by each partner

* abstinence

* rubbing your genitals on another person's thighs or belly or letting them do the same to you

* sucking or licking someone's nipples or unbroken skin

* rimming (anal–oral contact) with a dental dam

Research is showing that oral sex is riskier than previously thought. Much of HIV transmission has to do with infected bodily fluids coming into contact with open cuts and sores in the mouth. The best way to protect yourself during oral sex is with a latex condom (during fellatio) and with a dental dam or Saran Wrap (during cunnilingus).

Tip: Use water-based lube on the inside of these barriers to help with sensation. Don't use petroleum jelly, which can destroy latex.

If you're worried about getting HIV from giving oral sex, but absolutely won't use a barrier method, the next best thing to do is to not floss or brush your teeth for two hours before giving unprotected oral sex, to avoid creating tiny tears on the gumline and in the mouth. If you're worried about bad breath, or just want to freshen up, use Listerine or some other antibacterial mouthwash to take care of that problem.

So, Sexually, What *Can* I Do?

A lot of times when people talk about sex, especially HIV and sex, the conversation boils down to what we *can't* do or what we *shouldn't* do. Because this chapter shouldn't be completely negative, let's go over what you *can* do.

SAFER SEX ACTIVITIES

HIV transmission from the following activities is extremely unlikely:

- ✳ oral sex with a man who is wearing a condom

- ✳ oral sex with a woman using a dental dam or plastic wrap

- ✳ penile–vaginal intercourse **using a latex condom**, if the condom is used properly and doesn't break

- ✳ anal intercourse **using a latex condom**, if the condom is used properly and doesn't break

- ✳ sharing a sex toy and using a clean condom on it when switching the toy from one person's body to the other's

- ✳ monogamy—you and your partner have been tested, at both the beginning of sexual relations and three months later after the incubation period, are both HIV-negative, and from that point on *have sex only with each other* (if you and your partner want to be even more confident about your health status, you and your partner also get tested at six months after possible HIV exposure as well)

Signs and Symptoms of HIV/AIDS

After becoming infected with HIV, a person may not feel or look sick for years. Often, an HIV+ individual feels healthy and has no symptoms. In many cases, HIV lies dormant in a person's body for up to seven or nine years before its retrovirus effects are seen as symptoms. Flulike symptoms (chills, aches, fever) do appear early on for some people.

AIDS-related symptoms usually do develop in 70 to 80 percent of adults who have tested positive for HIV. Over time, the nervous and immune systems become damaged and HIV-infected people become sick with different illnesses.

> AIDS-Related Complex (ARC) or "lesser AIDS" is when one has a damaged immune system because of HIV exposure, but doesn't contract the opportunistic diseases that lead to a diagnosis of full-blown AIDS. ARC is often, but not always, fatal.

HOW CAN I TELL IF MY PARTNER OR I HAVE HIV?

You can't. The only way to find out is through an HIV test. So since you can't know if a person is HIV-free, and if you want to ease your mind about it, you may want to suggest that you and your partner get tested.

HIV Tests

HOW IS HIV DIAGNOSED?

HIV is diagnosed with an **HIV antibody test**. A sample of your blood is taken and sent to a lab to be tested for the presence of HIV antibodies. It usually takes two to three weeks for the test results to come back. Accurate testing for HIV antibodies takes so long because it requires two different tests. The screening test is the ELISA (Enzyme-Linked ImmunoSorben Assay) test. Positive ELISA tests are confirmed by a second test, either the Western Blot or the IFA (ImmunoFlourescent Assay) test.

You cannot get tested for HIV until at least twelve weeks—three months—after the time of possible exposure. During this time, often called the *"window period,"* antibodies will not appear in your blood, so it is useless to get tested if less than three months have passed since your time of possible exposure. Testing done before three months may not find an infection in some people and come up as a *"false negative."* The most reliable test results can be obtained six months after the last time you may have been exposed to the virus.

WHAT ARE THE POSSIBLE TEST RESULTS?

A **positive test result** means that you have been infected with HIV and that you can pass the virus on to others. You are HIV positive (HIV+). You have HIV in your blood and semen or vaginal fluid. Being HIV+ does not mean that you have AIDS or that you will necessarily develop AIDS.

A **negative test result** means that there were no HIV antibodies in your blood at the time of your test. You are HIV negative (HIV–). Being HIV– means that either you do not have an HIV infection or that you do have HIV infection but have not yet developed the antibodies for it. It doesn't mean that you're immune to the virus or that you cannot become infected in the future.

HIV tests are extremely accurate. The ELISA test can have a "false positive" or a "false negative" on occasion. (A false positive test is one that is positive even though the blood doesn't really contain HIV antibodies.) For this reason, the blood is tested a second time with the ELISA test and confirmed with a positive Western Blot or IFA to indicate a "positive test result."

HOW IS HIV/AIDS TREATED?

There is no cure for HIV infection or for AIDS. If you are diagnosed as HIV+, find yourself a knowledgeable, experienced, and supportive health-care provider to help you evaluate and manage your HIV infection. (There are drugs available that can help you to manage your infection—though not cure it—for years.) A health service or local AIDS community service organization will be able to give you a recommendation for such a provider. Take care of your body. Avoid alcohol and drugs since they can damage your immune system. Try to find some comfort and strength in a nutritious diet, stress reduction, restful sleep, regular exercise, and meditation.

SHOULD I GET TESTED?

You may be debating whether or not you should get tested. If you've put yourself at risk, it's a really good idea. If you haven't put yourself at risk, it's probably not necessary, but if you would like to put your mind at ease no matter what kind of sexual activity you've been participating in, then testing is a good idea.

In deciding if you've been at risk or if you should get tested, you should talk to a counselor at a test center or community-based HIV/AIDS service organization that provides test-counseling services. These people can help you make your decision and help you through the testing process if you decide to get tested.

If you do decide to get tested, do the following:

*   Get tested only at a center that offers both pre- and post-test counseling.

*   Get tested at a center where you don't have to give out your name or other personal information, like your social security number.

Getting tested for HIV can be a nerve-wracking experience, not so much because of the actual testing but because of the possible consequences. The test result could be something you may not want to deal with, or may not be psychologically prepared to deal with. While there can be a great deal of fear in getting tested and receiving positive test results, you need to get over your anxiety and effectively deal with the issues at hand. This is extremely important, because if you are HIV+, you need to prevent any complications and you need to delay the progress of the HIV infection. Plus, you need to make sure that you're not spreading the virus along to your partner(s). The earlier you seek treatment, the better.

While all of us need to be concerned about HIV, I hope that none of us have to deal with an HIV infection. The best way of coping with any concerns and fears you have is to avoid putting yourself at risk. Practice safer sex or don't have sex. It's that easy to stay healthy.

RESOURCES

For more information on HIV/AIDS, call or visit the following:

American Social Health Association—National AIDS Hotline: (800) 342-AIDS (342-2437) or www.ashastd.org

HIV/AIDS Treatment Information Service: (800) 448-0440

AZT Hotline at the National Institutes of Health: (800) 843-9388

Public Health Service Hotline: (800) 342-AIDS (342-2437)

AIDS Education Global Information System: www.aegis.com

CHAPTER 8

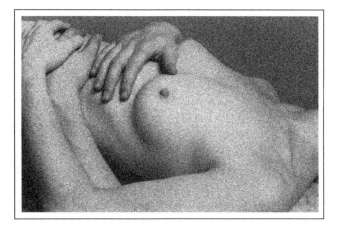

Gettin' Jiggy with Contraception:

The Bare Essentials of Pregnancy and STD Prevention

What are the different types of condoms?

What are polyurethane condoms?

What are the advantages/disadvantages of different contraceptive methods?

What do I do if I miss a day of the pill?

What are the signs of pregnancy?

When should I take an Emergency Contraceptive Pill?

Now that I've gotten you all stressed out about STDs and HIV, I'm sure that you'd love to know how to protect yourself from them. On top of that, you may have concerns about how to avoid the whole pregnancy thing. So now more than anything, we're going to ignite or rekindle that love affair every one of you should have with that trusty, close friend of ours—the condom—as well as cover other methods of contraception. This chapter is not only about making sure that you know how to protect yourself from STDs and HIV, but it is also about making sure that no little person is going to be calling you "Mommy" or "Daddy" anytime soon.

Modern contraceptives, or birth control, are among the greatest inventions we've seen in recent decades. Think about it—how many inventions do you know of, besides those coin-operated rocking horses outside of Wal-Mart, that allow you to hop in the saddle and become an uninhibited, untamed, giddy-up-and-go, worry-free rodeo rider?

Contraceptive Users

There are some young adults who have a good thing going on when they hit the sheets—they use contraceptives. What makes this group so appealing? According to a study done on how people who are effective and efficient users of contraceptives are viewed by others, contraceptive users are generally seen as mature, independent, self-reliant, secure, ambitious, decisive, and intelligent. They usually have a good self-image, assume responsibility with ease and confidence, carry accepted tasks through to completion, control their impulses, and have the capacity to tolerate frustration. They often establish and appreciate long-range goals and have a capacity to establish good communication and good sexual relationships with their partners.

Sven, a 23-year-old art enthusiast, explains his stance on contraceptives:

> I totally believe in using contraceptives, even though I don't necessarily like them. I don't think that it's worth the risk of contracting HIV or an STD or getting a girl pregnant. I got better at using contraceptives in college than in high school, when I did things I now regret. In youth, pleasure overrules commonsense. But now I realize that it's not worth the risks. I am a faithful condom user.

Nonusers of contraceptives, on the other hand, are characterized in general as immature, dependent, insecure, impulsive, and indecisive. They are said to have low self-esteem and little desire to control their lives or the world around them. They have limited ability to assume responsibility, to complete self-assumed tasks, to tolerate frustration, and to appreciate long-range goals.

Which way would you like to be described?

Choosing a Contraceptive

Deciding on a contraceptive method is no easy matter. Whether it's a barrier method, hormonal method, or family planning technique, there are so many choices! It's a huge decision, one that's based on your current state of health, lifestyle, beliefs, and sexual activity. It may take some research to select the form of contraception that's best for you, and that is what this chapter is for—to help you determine which contraceptive(s) you'd like to be the most dependent upon. In deciding upon a method, remember that condoms are the best method available in protecting you against both pregnancy and STDs/HIV.

Other than abstinence, no method of birth control is 100 percent effective at preventing conception. Yet, there are a number of safe and effective methods to choose from that are almost 100 percent effective. In choosing one, ask yourself the following questions:

* How does my partner feel about birth control?

* Is this method easy to use? How likely am I to use it?

✳ How often do I have sex? Do I want a method that's always in my body?

✳ Do I need a method that helps to protect me from STDs and HIV?

✳ What are the health risks associated with this method?

✳ Do I have religious or moral feelings about using birth control? Which methods fit with my religious beliefs?

✳ Will I feel embarrassed about using this method?

✳ How much will this method cost? Can I afford it?

✳ How do I feel about touching my body in order to use this method?

HOW DOES A FEMALE GET PREGNANT?

It would be helpful to know how a woman becomes pregnant before deciding upon a contraceptive method. Every twenty-one to forty days, a woman usually has her period. In between periods, the woman **ovulates**— her body releases an egg. If during this time the egg meets up with any sperm that may be in her reproductive system due to sexual relations, it may become fertilized and eventually implant itself into the female's uterus. If a sperm does not fertilize the egg, the egg leaves the female's body and she has her period.

A woman is most likely to get pregnant around the time of her ovulation, which usually takes place sometime between the week after her period and the week before her period. However, this isn't always the case. Sometimes a woman's period is not that regular and ovulation can happen at any time during her cycle, even during her period. So a woman can get pregnant at any point of her cycle—*even during the week of her period.*

> The most common physical risk associated with unprotected sex is pregnancy, with the likelihood of pregnancy resulting from any single unprotected act of vaginal intercourse being one in seventy. About six out of every ten pregnancies in the United States are unplanned and 85 percent of women who use no contraception during vaginal intercourse become pregnant each year.

Barrier Methods of Contraception (Nonhormonal Contraceptives)

Barrier methods are those contraceptives that block sperm from traveling past the cervix and into the uterus. They offer pregnancy protection without the risk of hormonal side effects. The condom is the most effective of the barrier methods, making it my personal favorite and the reason why I spend more time on it in this chapter than on any other contraceptive. The condom is tops because, in preventing sperm from being deposited into the vagina, anus, or mouth, it greatly reduces the risk of pregnancy and/or STD/HIV transmission. Condoms are your ticket to safer sex.

THE MALE CONDOM

What Is It?

An impermeable sheath worn over an *erect* penis is the best way, other than refraining from sexual intercourse, to protect yourself against sexually transmitted infections. A condom can be made of latex, plastic, or animal tissue, and it catches semen before, during, and after ejaculation. It prevents the spread of disease by keeping vaginal and anal mucous membranes from coming into contact with both the penis and the semen. Some condoms have a nipple-shaped tip to hold the semen, others do not.

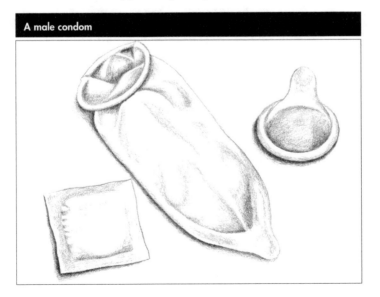

A male condom

Note: In order for you and your partner to get the maximum possible protection from a condom, you have to know how to *properly* put it on *every single time* you have sexual relations. It is essential to follow the steps below to make sure your condom protects you and your partner. If you practice these steps a couple of times on your own, pretty soon you'll be whipping on this party hat in record time, hardly interrupting the heat of the moment.

Using a Condom Properly

1. Make sure you have a trusted brand.

2. Check the expiration date (ahead of time if possible).

3. Make sure the condom is right side out.

4. Use a reservoir-tip condom, or pinch a half-inch at the tip. (This leaves some space for the semen to be collected.)

5. If the penis isn't circumcised, pull back the foreskin before rolling on the condom.

6. Pinch the air out of the tip with one hand and be

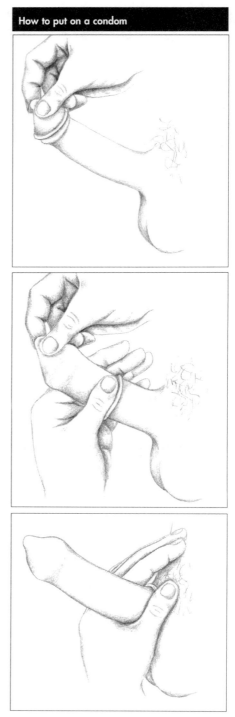

How to put on a condom

careful not to use your nails. (Note: Friction against air bubbles can cause a condom to break.)

7. Put the condom on the erect penis, before the penis makes first contact with the vagina, anus, or mouth, and slowly and carefully unroll the condom all the way down the shaft of the penis, smoothing out air bubbles.

8. After ejaculation, withdraw while the penis is still erect and remove the condom carefully, holding onto the base to prevent slipping. Be careful not to spill the contents.

9. Wrap the condom in tissue and throw it in the trash. Don't flush it down the toilet since that could cause plumbing problems!

Possible Side Effects

* None, unless either partner has a latex allergy.

Effectiveness

When used properly and consistently, latex condoms used *with* a spermicide are about 98 to 99 percent effective. They rarely break. Among the different types of condoms, "extra strength" condoms are actually no better than "regular" or "thin" condoms when it comes to effectiveness. Latex condoms offer good protection against gonorrhea, chlamydia, syphilis, HIV, pelvic inflammatory disease, and vaginitis. Latex condoms offer *some* protection against HPV, herpes, and hepatitis B. In offering some protection against HPV, they also reduce a woman's chances of getting cervical cancer.

Spermicidally lubricated condoms are unlikely to be more effective than regular condoms in the prevention of pregnancy, since they don't provide enough spermicide to do the job effectively. If you'd like to use spermicide, I recommend that you apply additional amounts on your own. This is actually a great idea, since without spermicide a condom's efficacy rate drops to 88 percent, with 12 out of every 100 women who use this contraceptive for one year becoming pregnant. This percentage is also mostly due to the condoms not being used consistently or correctly.

Out of 100 couples who use condoms correctly and consistently for one year, only three couples will experience an accidental pregnancy.

COUNTLESS CONDOMS!

One cool thing about using condoms is that you have such a wide array of different types of condoms to choose from. In shopping for condoms, you can feel like a kid in a candy store once again—excited and overwhelmed by the many tempting choices. *Condomania!!!* Choosing which style of condoms to use can be quite a dilemma at first, but a fun one at that. One way to solve that "problem" is to simply try them all and see which one you and your partner like best!

Styles of Condoms

* lubricated or nonlubricated
* with or without spermicide
* reservoir tip—generally easier to use
* ribbed or smooth
* flavored
* extra-sensitive
* polyurethane
* lambskin—(I don't recommend these condoms since they are expensive and do not protect from HIV and other viruses.)

Once you've decided on the type of condom you're going to use for your next wild and crazy—yet safer—sexual encounter, you'll want to make sure that you're getting the most satisfying and erotic protection out of your condoms. You always want to be prepared for the worst kind of weather. So in order for your condoms to give you and your partner nothing but the best, you'll want to keep some of the following tips in mind:

Tips for Using Condoms

* Don't keep your condoms in your pocket, glove compartment, or wallet for weeks, or in the sun—heat makes them more likely to break. Store your condoms at a temperature of 50° to 85°F.

* For maximum effectiveness for birth control, condoms should be used with a spermicidal foam or cream.

✳ Be sure to leave some space at the tip for ejaculate.

✳ Do not reuse condoms.

✳ Place a dab of gel-like lubricant, like K-Y Jelly, in the tip of the condom before rolling it down the penis for *added sensation* during sex. The lube causes the condom to rub against the penis during sex, creating a smooth, stimulating friction!

✳ If you're using a condom for oral sex, make sure it's unlubricated and without spermicide. Nothing spoils fellatio like the taste of nonoxynol-9.

✳ Never use an oil-based lubricant, such as Vaseline, baby oil, or skin lotions, because these substances will weaken the latex condom and cause it to deteriorate.

✳ Put the condom on before the penis touches the vulva, anus, or mouth. Pre-ejaculate can carry enough sperm to cause pregnancy or to spread an STD.

✳ Look for a date of manufacture on the condom, and do not use it if it is more than five years old. If you can't find a date of manufacture, don't use it at all!

Most condom users carry their condoms around with them. The persons most likely to carry condoms are young, single males. Among users, 70 percent of men and 56 percent of women carry condoms on them.

COMBATING CONDOM CRITICS

People have a lot of beliefs about condoms. Some are afraid that using condoms makes sex seem premeditated rather than spontaneous, that it reduces the pleasure of vaginal or anal intercourse and romance, and that it makes sex unnatural. Some people believe that using a condom will offend their partner and that purchasing condoms is embarrassing and inconvenient. To top it off, a lot of this thinking is rationalized with the belief that treatments for STDs are easily available, so prevention is not an issue. And then there is the belief that condoms might not be that reliable or effective. I beg to differ on all of those.

Condoms are an excellent enhancement to your sexual escapades, because they are meant to protect you and your partner—keep each of you healthy, and healthy together, at that. Condoms can put a damper on sex only if you let them. You have control over your attitude toward condoms. You can eroticize condom use.

Personally, I can't think of anything that's sexier and brings more relief when fooling around than a partner whipping out a condom. First, the cue that you're going to get some is hot. Second, it tells you that your partner cares about and respects you and your health. What could be more erotic than that? It always feels good to know that someone is looking out for you, that they're on your team.

With positive thinking and the willingness to experiment with condoms and acknowledge all of the rewards your sexual relationship could reap from using them, you will, I hope, forget that you ever had any of those negative beliefs. If you need a boost in positive condom thinking from time to time, consider me your condom cheerleader. Below are some advantages to condoms to cheer you on.

Advantages

- are easy to use, buy, and carry

- are used only when needed

- are relatively inexpensive ($1.35 for three condoms)

- mean that responsibility is shared by both partners

- can be used as a back-up for other contraceptive methods

- can help maintain an erection

- can help relieve premature ejaculation

- provide the best protection available against STDs and HIV

- do not create hormonal side effects

- have no serious side effects or impacts on one's future ability to bear children

- reduce a woman's chances of getting cervical cancer, as they offer some protection against HPV

Now that I've gotten you all psyched up about condoms, I have to admit that they do have a few drawbacks.

Disadvantages

- ✳ may not protect from all STDs—certain sexual practices, like grinding, may place you at a high risk for certain STDs, such as HPV, herpes, and hepatitis, even if you use a condom (see Chapter 6 for more on STDs and how they are transmitted and see pages 122–123 for descriptions of high-, low-, and no-risk sexual behaviors as they relate to the transmission of HIV)

- ✳ must be put on during sex

- ✳ can break or slip off during sex

- ✳ may cause an allergic reaction

- ✳ are ineffective if used *incorrectly*

- ✳ may cause decreased sensation for men

- ✳ spermicide-lubricated condoms may irritate the vagina or penis

Be sure to check every now and then to see that your condom hasn't slipped off!

How Do I Know Whether I'm Allergic to Latex?

In men, a condom allergy is usually easy to diagnose since the most common symptom is a rash in the genital area soon after intercourse. Women experience genital area itching and burning after exposure to latex condoms, and sometimes mistake such allergy symptoms for a recurrent yeast infection. A physician can help you determine if you have a latex allergy.

The chance that you're allergic to latex condoms is about 1 in 100.

Cost

Nonlubricated condoms start at $0.25; lubricated at $0.50; and textured at $2.50. Some university health centers and family planning clinics give them away.

Where Can You Get Them?

Condoms are available at drugstores, clinics, restroom vending machines, convenience stores, some supermarkets, and university health centers.

POLYURETHANE CONDOMS

What Is It?

Some condoms are made from plastic instead of rubber (e.g., Avanti by Durex and Trojan Supra). These are a terrific alternative for couples who are allergic to latex. Many couples are also finding that polyurethane condoms can spice up their sex lives. These condoms are preferred by most men over standard latex condoms because they are thinner and allow for increased sensation for both partners.

Effectiveness

Polyurethane condoms have a failure rate of anywhere from 4.4 to 15 percent. They break almost four times as often as the latex variety, mostly because of their reduced elasticity, and they slip off six times more often during intercourse. The research is still out on their effectiveness against pregnancy, STDs, and HIV. There are, however, no pores or holes in polyurethane, so even particles as small as sperm and the HIV virus should not be able to pass through this material. Polyurethane condoms have all the advantages of latex condoms plus those below.

Advantages

* are thinner—so most men feel more sensation, partly because polyurethane reportedly transmits more heat

* have a looser fit—so they're more comfortable for many men

* are colorless (transparent) and odorless

* don't taste bad if used for oral sex

* can be used with any type of lubricant, either oil- or water-based

* are more stable and will last longer than latex

* are perfect for people who are allergic to latex

Disadvantages

- ✳ have less elasticity than latex condoms, so they're more likely to break or slip off during use

- ✳ are twice the price of latex condoms

- ✳ are of inconsistent quality

Cost

You'll pay about $7 for six polyurethane condoms

Where Can You Get Them?

Polyurethane condoms are available at some drugstores, clinics, convenience stores, supermarkets, and university health centers.

> Make sure you change your condom if you're having an extra-long sex session. Condoms can wear out if you're at it for a really long time.

SHEEPSKIN CONDOMS

What Is It?

Though its name implies otherwise, this condom is made out of lamb intestines. It is good for protection against pregnancy only, but *not* against STDs and HIV. This condom has little pores in it that may allow small viruses, like HIV or hepatitis, to be transmitted. People sometimes prefer this condom because it "feels more natural" and because you can use any type of lubricant with it. For people with latex allergies, sheepskin condoms are better than no protection at all. However, they are also expensive, with a dozen costing as much as $20.

Where Can You Get Them?

Sheepskin condoms are available at some drugstores.

> "Novelty condoms" are those edible or specialty condoms often found in sex shops, adult bookstores, or in condom machines in public restrooms. They are not good for protection against HIV, STDs, or pregnancy. As their label, "For Novelty Use Only" implies, they are just for kicks.

SPERMICIDES

What Are They?

Spermicides are sperm-killing chemicals available as foam, cream, jelly, tablets, suppositories, or film. If placed in the vagina before intercourse, spermicides provide a physical barrier by blocking the sperm from entering the uterus, and kill sperm on contact by destroying sperm cell membranes.

Possible Side Effect

* * may cause an allergic reaction

> Nonoxynol-9, a common spermicide, is known to cause an increase in urinary tract infections (UTIs). It does so by increasing the production of candida bacteria that ascend into the bladder. UTI symptoms include painful urination, frequent urination, and pain in the urethra.

Effectiveness

When used with condoms *consistently* and *correctly* each time you have sex, spermicides can be up to 99 percent effective. Used alone, spermicides are much less effective—about 80 percent. Based on recent findings, the CDC no longer recommends spermicides, particularly Nonoxynol-9, as effective against organisms causing gonorrhea, syphilis, herpes, and trichomoniasis, as previously believed. For women with a vaginal sensitivity to Nonoxynol-9, the spermicide is thought to actually increase their vulnerability to HIV.

Advantages

* * are easy to buy and have handy
* * are easy to use and carry
* * can be used only when needed
* * have no serious hormonal side effects, nor any impact on future ability to bear children

Disadvantages

* * can produce genital irritations due to allergic reactions
* * may interrupt sex since it must be inserted before every act of sexual intercourse

* may be messy

* may produce an unpleasant smell

* provide short-lasting protection

Cost

Applicator kits of foam and gel cost $8 to $18; refills cost $4 to $8; films and suppositories are similarly priced.

Where Can You Get It?

Spermicides are available at drugstores, supermarkets, and clinics.

THE FEMALE CONDOM

What Is It?

The female condom is a plastic pouch, about 7 inches long and 3 inches wide, worn inside the vagina. It is a lubricated, polyurethane sheath, resembling a clear balloon, with a flexible, plastic ring at each end, and is marketed under the brand name Reality. It's inserted before intercourse and catches semen. The ring at the closed end is used for insertion. A woman puts it in, like a tampon, until it is resting firmly behind her pubic bone. The open-end ring stays on the outside of the body and lies flat against the vaginal entrance to hold the sheath in place. It is removed immediately after sex, before the woman stands up. The outer ring is squeezed together and twisted to keep semen inside.

> Do not use this condom in addition to a regular male condom!! The friction caused by the two layers of protection rubbing against each other could cause breakage.

Possible Side Effect

* can result in vaginal or penile irritation (from spermicide)

Effectiveness

Female condoms have a higher failure rate than male latex condoms. Of couples using these condoms consistently and correctly, 5 percent will become pregnant.

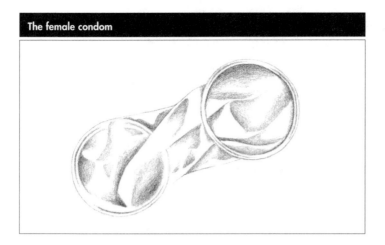

The female condom

Advantages

- ✱ can be used by people with latex allergies

- ✱ can be left in place for as long as you like after sex—maintaining the spontaneity of the moment

- ✱ gives the female more control because she uses a contraceptive at her discretion

- ✱ protects against STDs and HIV

- ✱ is less susceptible to tearing and doesn't deteriorate with exposure to oil-based substances

- ✱ doesn't require a doctor to get it

- ✱ can be inserted hours in advance

- ✱ is made of polyurethane, which transmits heat well

- ✱ creates no serious medical or hormonal side effects, nor any impact on future ability to bear children

Disadvantages

- ✱ gets in the way of manual or oral stimulation

- ✱ not ideal for wearing out during an evening before sex

- ✱ can be noisy

- ✱ is three times more expensive than male condoms

Cost

Female condoms cost about $3 each and are usually sold in packs of three.

Where Can You Get It?

You can get female condoms at drugstores and at some clinics.

THE CONTRACEPTIVE SPONGE

What Is It?

The sponge is a soft, polyurethane foam device, shaped like a donut, containing the spermicide Nonoxynol-9. It fits over the cervix, and blocks and kills sperm moving toward the uterus. Before intercourse, the woman wets the sponge to activate the spermicide. She then inserts the sponge into her vagina far enough back to cover her cervix. There, it will absorb sperm and also block it from entering the cervix. It must be left in place for at least six hours after sex. A woven polyester loop is designed to ease removal.

How Is It Used?

The sponge is moistened and inserted into the vagina up to an hour before intercourse and may be left in place for up to twenty-four hours.

Possible Side Effects

* irritation

* vaginal discharge

* allergic reaction

* Toxic Shock Syndrome (TSS)—in very rare cases, there is an increased risk for TSS if sponge is left in for longer than thirty hours at a time

Effectiveness

Generally, the sponge has an 80 percent effectiveness rate for women who have never borne children. It is *not* effective against STDs and HIV.

Advantages

* is easy to buy and have handy

* is usually easy to insert

* does not require separate application of spermicide

* may be inserted ahead of time to allow for sexual spontaneity

* is available at a pharmacy without a prescription

Disadvantages

* *doesn't protect against any STDs or HIV*

* cannot be reused after removal

* may be difficult to insert or remove on occasion

* requires that clean water be available for insertion

* cannot be used for short time after childbirth, abortion, or miscarriage, or when you have vaginal bleeding, your period, or any abnormal vaginal discharge

Cost

Each sponge costs about $2.

Where Can You Get It?

The sponge has not been available since 1995 when it was taken off the market because of production problems, but the sponge is coming back!!! It should be available in U.S. drugstores soon and is already available in Canada.

THE DIAPHRAGM

What Is It?

A diaphragm is a small, flexible rubber (latex) dome that fits inside the vagina over the cervix. The diaphragm may be inserted up to six hours before intercourse, and with spermicide helps to block and kill sperm moving toward the uterus. It must not be removed until at least six hours after the last ejaculation. The spermicide *must* be smeared on the inside cup of the diaphragm—the side that faces up. After this has been done, fold the diaphragm in half and insert it into the vagina, where it will unfold and lie against the cervix. In order for it to work properly, the woman must be fitted for her diaphragm before she uses it for the first time.

Effectiveness

This method is about 82 to 94 percent effective. Its failure rate is mostly due to improper use. It's *not* effective against most STDs or HIV, due to the fact that semen is deposited directly into the vagina and it allows skin-on-skin contact.

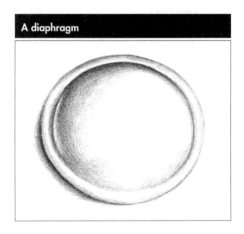

A diaphragm

Possible Side Effects

✳ allergic reactions

✳ Urinary Tract (bladder) Infections (UTIs)

✳ Toxic Shock Syndrome (TSS)—in very rare cases, there is increased risk if diaphragm is left in for longer than twenty-four hours at a time

Advantages

✳ usually has no serious medical side effects or impact on future ability to bear children

✳ may be inserted up to two hours ahead of time to allow for sexual spontaneity

✳ can last for years

Disadvantages

* *doesn't protect against any STDs or HIV*

* requires a medical exam and periodic professional refitting

* requires professional instruction about insertion and removal

* requires a backup contraceptive until use is mastered

* may become dislodged

* may cause allergy, to latex and/or spermicide

* increases risk of bladder infection

* for some women, it is hard to put in and take out

* cannot be used for a short time after childbirth, abortion, miscarriage, or when you are having vaginal bleeding, including your periods, or any abnormal vaginal discharge

* may be messy because of repeated insertions of contraceptive jelly or cream

* must be left in place six to eight hours after sex

* may cause repeated UTIs that persist despite efforts to refit diaphragm

* must be refitted if you gain or lose ten pounds

Cost

A diaphragm costs $13 to $25, with the fitting and examination costing about $50 to $125.

Where Can You Get It?

You can get fitted for a diaphragm at a doctor's office or family health clinic.

You will know you have a urinary tract infection (UTI), which is due to bacteria being trapped inside your urethra, if you experience a burning sensation during urination; have cloudy, odorous urine; and experience the urgency to urinate frequently. UTIs are common in women who are sexually active with a new partner. A UTI can be cured with antibiotics. Meanwhile, you should drink lots of cranberry juice and water, and urinate after you have sex.

CERVICAL CAP

What Is It?

The cervical cap is a small, thimble-shaped, latex rubber cup that fits snugly over the cervix and stays in place by suction. It can be worn for up to forty-eight hours and should remain in place for eight hours after intercourse. The cap has a small groove in its inner surface that allows it to attach itself by suction to the cervix. It is then able to prevent sperm from moving past the cervix and into the uterus. The cap is inserted before intercourse and *must* be used with spermicides, which kill the sperm. Spermicides should be carefully applied prior to intercourse so that they do not interfere with the seal created by the cap.

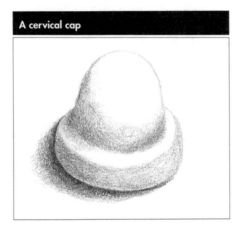

A cervical cap

Effectiveness

In women who have not had a child, the cervical cap is 82 to 91 percent effective. For women who have had a child, the effectiveness rate is 64 to 74 percent.

Possible Side Effects

* ✳ cervical irritation
* ✳ Toxic Shock Syndrome (TSS)—in very rare cases, there is increased risk if cap is left in for more than forty-eight hours at a time
* ✳ Urinary Tract Infections (UTIs)

Advantages

* can be left in place longer than other contraceptive methods, and additional contraceptive cream or jelly isn't needed for repeated sexual intercourse during that time

* not associated with any major health concerns

* can last for several years

* has no serious medical or hormonal side effects or impact on future ability to bear children

Disadvantages

* *provides no protection against STDs and HIV*

* may lead to abnormal Pap smears and unpleasant odors and discharge if left in too long

* requires planning

* can be messy

* can cause allergies, to latex and/or spermicide

* cannot be used during vaginal bleeding or infection

* may be difficult to fit for some women, since it comes in only four sizes

* may increase UTIs

Cost

Cervical caps cost about $13 to $25, with an examination and a fitting running $50 to $125.

Where Can You Get It?

Go to a doctor's office or family health clinic to be fitted for a cervical cap.

Hormonal Contraception Methods

ORAL CONTRACEPTIVES

So maybe you (and your partner) have decided that you're not at great risk for getting an STD and don't want to use condoms, or maybe you want extra protection against pregnancy, in addition to a barrier method, when you're messing around. Among your many choices is the method of contraception that sixteen million American women and sixty million women worldwide use—the birth control pill!

Oral contraceptives, popularly referred to as "the Pill," are the most popular form of reversible contraception in the United States. Combination pills, which contain the hormones estrogen and progestin, are the most commonly prescribed oral contraceptive. Minipills, which only contain progestin, are usually prescribed only to women who should not take estrogen.

When the pill first came out back in the 1960s, it revolutionized the sex lives of women everywhere. With such a high rate of effectiveness, women could finally relax when fooling around, knowing that the chances of getting pregnant were slim. Soon, women were able to tune into their inner sex diva and let loose during sex—start to truly enjoy it. Pill users to this day claim to have this same unleashing of enthusiasm and sexual energy due to the fact that they're on the pill and are free from concerns about pregnancy.

> While oral contraceptives are great protection against pregnancy, condoms give you the best protection against both pregnancy and STDs/HIV when you're fooling around.

THE COMBINATION PILL

What Is It?

As mentioned above, combination pills contain hormones that are similar to hormones that regulate the menstrual cycle. A woman takes the pills for either twenty-one or twenty-eight days each month to prevent pregnancy. The hormones in the pills stop the egg from being released every month. They also make the cervical mucus thicker in order to stop sperm from getting into the uterus. A woman takes one pill a day, regardless of whether or not she plans to have sex that day.

There are more than twenty brands of oral contraceptives available, each with different strengths and combinations of hormones, mostly estrogen and progestin. Besides being used for birth control, oral contraceptives have historically been prescribed for androgen disorders, menorrhagia (excessive menstrual flow), acne, endometriosis, dysfunctional uterine bleeding, and menstrual irregularities. It is the most popular contraceptive method used today.

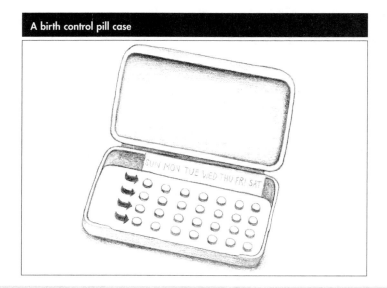

A birth control pill case

What If I Miss a Day?

If you miss just one day, take your pill as soon as you remember to take it and take the next pill at your regular time, even if it means taking two pills on the same day. If you forget to take your pill for two or more days, take two pills the day you remember and two pills the next day. Then take one pill per day until you finish the pack. Remember that nearly seven million women worldwide have unintended pregnancies every year because they fail to take their birth control pill correctly.

Effectiveness

Used correctly, the pill is effective 97 to 99 percent of the time. The Pill's effectiveness may be reduced if the woman is taking medications, such as certain antibiotics. It is *not* effective against STDs or HIV.

Possible Side Effects

Many of the side effects listed below often disappear within the first few months of using the Pill. If they do not, a woman should consult her doctor and ask to get put on a different type of pill.

   ✳   nausea

   ✳   fluid retention

   ✳   weight gain or loss

✳ breast tenderness

✳ missed periods

✳ spotting between periods

✳ vaginal infections

✳ headaches

✳ increased amounts of vaginal discharge

✳ susceptibility to vaginitis, because the Pill alters the chemical balance of the lining of the vagina

✳ mood changes, irritability, and/or depression

✳ increases in certain diseases of the circulatory system, such as heart disease

✳ benign liver tumors (if a woman takes the Pill for more than five years)

As many women lose weight as gain weight while on oral contraceptive pills.

Advantages

✳ is easy to use

✳ doesn't interrupt sex and spontaneity

✳ reduces PMS tension and cramps

✳ reduces amount of menstrual flow (by up to 60 percent)

✳ may make menstrual periods less painful and more regular

✳ reduces menstrual cramping, acne, spotting, iron deficiency anemia, and premenstrual tension

✳ may lower chances of getting pelvic inflammatory disease (PID); ovarian cysts (by 80 to 90 percent); cancer of the ovaries, endometrium, and uterus; noncancerous breast tumors; and anemia

✳ lowers number of future tubal (ectopic) pregnancies

Disadvantages

* *doesn't protect against any STDs or HIV*

* may make user more susceptible to chlamydia and gonorrhea

* is expensive

* places the entire burden of contraception on the woman

* requires a medical exam and prescription

* must be taken on a regular schedule—daily

* is less effective when taken with certain drugs

* increases metabolism of some drugs, making them more potent

* may result in spotting during first few cycles

* may lead to depression, fatigue, mood changes, and anxiety

* may be difficult for some women to get pregnant for several months after stopping use

* is not recommended for women who smoke, especially those over 35 years of age

The risk of death for women over age 35 who smoke and use the Pill is much higher than for nonsmokers. They are ten times more likely to have a heart attack than women who don't smoke or take the Pill. This is especially true among women who have diabetes, high blood pressure, or elevated cholesterol. If she's a smoker, a woman needs to choose between kicking the habit or going on the Pill.

Cost
Monthly pill packs are $15 to $25, but cost less if obtained at clinics. A visit to a physician for an initial exam can be $25 to $135, although some family planning clinics charge patients according to income.

Where Can You Get It?
You must go to a doctor or a health clinic to get a prescription.

MINIPILLS

What Are They?

Minipills are birth control pills that contains only the hormone progestin. They are designed to avoid the estrogen-related side effects of standard pills. No one is exactly sure how minipills work. It is thought that they work by reducing and thickening cervical mucus to prevent sperm from reaching the egg. The pills also keep the uterine lining from thickening, which prevents a fertilized egg from implanting in the uterus.

Effectiveness

These are slightly less effective than the combination pill—a typical-user failure rate is 2.5 percent. The failure rate increases in women who weigh over 154 pounds. Since the dosage is smaller, minipill users have to be diligent about taking this pill at the *same time* every day. Minipills have the greatest effectiveness when a woman's "normal" bleeding pattern is most irregular. Minipills become effective anywhere from seven to twenty-eight days after a woman begins taking them. They are *not* effective against STDs or HIV.

Possible Side Effects

 * changes in menstrual cycle

 * weight gain

 * breast tenderness

 * irregular bleeding

 * tubal (ectopic) pregnancy

Advantages

 * can decrease menstrual bleeding and cramps

 * decreases risk of pelvic inflammatory disease (PID), and endometrial and ovarian cancer

Disadvantages

 * the same as for the regular birth control pill

Where Can You Get It?

You must go to a doctor or a health clinic to get a prescription.

INTRAUTERINE DEVICE (IUD)

What Is It?

An IUD is a small piece of plastic, about an inch long, in the shape of a "T" or "7," that is placed in the uterus. It has a monofilament string so that a woman can check to make sure that the IUD is in place. There are two types of IUDs available in the United States: the Copper T-380A (also known as ParaGuard), and Progestasert Progesterone T. No one is completely sure how the IUD works. Experts think that the copper of the IUD, or the hormones that some IUDs release, interfere with sperm movement, stop sperm from reaching the egg, and change the lining of the uterus so that a woman will not get pregnant. It may do this by causing an inflammatory response to foreign objects in the uterus, creating an influx of white blood cells that kill off egg-seeking sperm. The latest copper IUD is indicated for ten years of use. The Progestasert IUD needs to be replaced about once a year because of its daily release of synthetic hormone progesterone.

How Is It Used?

A clinician inserts the IUD into the uterus through a straight narrow tube. Insertion takes only about five minutes and is performed during or immediately after your period. You need only to check its placement after each period. The IUD may be removed by a health-care professional at any time.

Effectiveness

An IUD is 97.4 to 99.2 percent effective. Two out of every hundred women who use an IUD for one year will get pregnant. The IUD is effective immediately upon insertion. Some women who use an IUD may expel it by normal uterine contractions during the first year, though expulsion is most likely to occur during the first three months. It is not effective against STDs or HIV.

The IUD is the world's second-most popular female contraceptive, used by 13 percent of all women of reproductive age, although only 1 percent of

American women use it. Anybody can use the IUD, although it is best suited for women with families. Women who have multiple sex partners or have reproductive abnormalities, active or recent pelvic infections, anemia, heavy menstrual or abnormal vaginal bleeding, or past tubal pregnancies are not good candidates for the IUD.

Why do so few people in the United States use the IUD? Back in the early 1970s, Dalkon Shield's IUD was pulled off the market by the U.S. Food and Drug Administration. It appeared to have a design flaw in its "tail" that tended to draw bacteria from the vagina into the uterus, resulting in infection in some women. Although the problem has been corrected, women here have been a little wary of the IUD ever since.

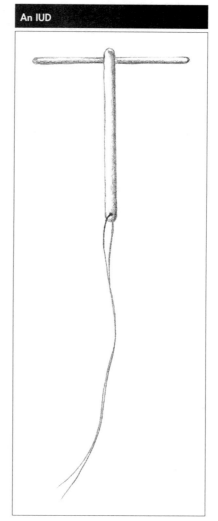

An IUD

Possible Side Effects

✳ increased menstrual flow, cramps, or backaches— (significantly reduced if using Progestasert)

✳ spotting between periods

✳ heavier and longer periods

✳ allergic reaction to copper (very rare)

✳ mild bleeding and pain

✳ increased risk of pelvic inflammatory disease (PID) and tubal infection

✳ increased chance of tubal (ectopic) pregnancy

Advantages

* does not interfere with sexual spontaneity

* requires no daily attention

* the Copper T-380 IUD can be left in place for up to ten years

* largely eliminates human error

* is comfortable—you should not be able to feel it is there

* may reduce menstrual cramps (IUDs with hormones)

Disadvantages

* *does not protect against STDs or HIV*

* may be uncomfortable during insertion

* may make users more susceptible to chlamydia and gonorrhea

* requires a medical exam

* is not offered at many student health centers

* may make it hard for you to ever become pregnant

* can puncture the womb

* must be taken out if you become pregnant

Cost

An IUD costs approximately $100 to $300. Insertion fees run from $160 to $400. Some family planning clinics charge according to income.

Where Can You Get It?

You can get an IUD from your doctor or at some health clinics.

DEPO-PROVERA

What Is It?

Depo-Provera is an injection that uses a synthetic hormone, progestin (as in the birth control pill), to prevent pregnancy. The hormone makes the cervical mucus thicker so it's harder for the sperm to enter the womb, and it may also stop eggs from leaving the ovary. Depo-Provera inhibits ovulation, thickens cervical mucus, and inhibits growth of the endometrium so that the fertilized egg is unable to implant itself. The injection is given in the upper arm or in the buttocks, and while most women say that it isn't very painful, the injection site may be slightly sore for a day or so. Depo-Provera is used in over 80 countries.

How Often Do You Get an Injection?

Depo-Provera is injected once every thirteen weeks—four times a year.

Effectiveness

Depo-Provera is 99.7 percent effective, as long as you remember to get your injection once every three months. In order for Depo-Provera to become effective immediately after the injection, you must receive your first injection during the first five days of a normal menstrual period. If you don't get the shot during that time period, you have to wait five days after your shot for it to become effective, and you should use a backup method during sex. It is *not* effective against STDs or HIV.

Possible Side Effects

* weight gain/bloating

* irregular or unpredictable menstrual bleeding

* heavier or lighter bleeding than normal for you during your period

* after one year, you may stop having periods altogether (amenorrhea)

* nervousness

* dizziness

* stomach discomfort

* breast swelling or tenderness

* headaches

* fatigue

* depression

* loss of interest in sex

* hair loss

* possible increase in chance of breast cancer

* possible association with decrease in amount of minerals stored in your bones, which can be considered among the risk factors for osteoporosis

Advantages

* has to be dealt with only four times a year

* doesn't interfere with sex

* reduces menstrual cramps

* decreases blood loss during periods

* lasts three months

* protects against cancer of the lining of the uterus and iron deficiency anemia

Disadvantages

* *doesn't offer any protection against STDs and HIV*

* must be injected by health-care provider

* may take up to a year to conceive after stopping injections

* increases risk of osteoporosis due to depletion of stored minerals in bones

* may lower woman's interest in sex if periods stop

Cost

Depo-Provera costs about the same per year as the birth control pill, with an injection costing $30 to $75; it may cost less at clinics. An examination will cost $35 to $125, with some family planning clinics charging according to income.

Where Can You Get It?

Doctors and some health clinics offer Depo-Provera.

LUNELLE

What Is It?

Lunelle is a combination of the hormones progestin and estrogen administered via a shot into a muscle every month. It prevents the release of the eggs during ovulation and prevents the lining of the uterus from preparing for a pregnancy.

Effectiveness

Lunelle has a failure rate of 0.2 to 0.4 percent. One in 200 to 400 women who use this method for a year will get pregnant.

Possible Side Effects

- ✳ breast tenderness
- ✳ changes in menstrual periods

Advantages

- ✳ doesn't interfere with sex
- ✳ doesn't cause a loss of bone density
- ✳ results in less weight gain than Depo-Provera
- ✳ needs to be dealt with only once per month
- ✳ allows for fertility to return soon after discontinuing use

Disadvantages

- ✳ *does not protect against STDs or HIV*
- ✳ may be inconvenient due to monthly shot
- ✳ causes changes in menstrual cycle, e.g., irregular bleeding
- ✳ cannot be used if breastfeeding

Cost

Lunelle costs $12 to $35 per month; plus $35 to $125 for the initial exam.

Where Can You Get It?

Health centers, family planning clinics, and physician's offices offer the exam and shots.

NORPLANT

What Is It?

Norplant is a set of six matchstick-sized, progestin hormone–containing capsules, made of silicone-based tubing (a soft, flexible material), that are inserted just beneath the skin of your upper inner arm. These capsules are implanted through a small incision just below the surface of the skin in a fan-shaped configuration. Norplant provides protection against pregnancy for up to five years. You are protected from pregnancy by the progestin levonorgestrel, which is slowly released from each capsule into the bloodstream twenty-four hours after the capsules are in place. The hormone makes the cervical mucus thicker so that it is hard for sperm to enter the womb. It may also stop eggs from leaving the ovary.

Effectiveness

Norplant is an amazing 99.96 percent effective. If it is inserted in the first seven days of a woman's menstrual cycle, it is immediately effective. It is *not* effective against STDs or HIV.

Possible Side Effects

✳ tenderness and bruising at insertion site for a couple of days

✳ irregular periods or spotting for 70 percent of women

✳ increased number of days of menstrual bleeding

✳ no period for many months *(amenorrhea)*

✳ breast tenderness

✳ headaches

✳ mood swings and/or depression

✳ nervousness

✳ dizziness

✳ weight gain

✳ hair loss

✳ acne

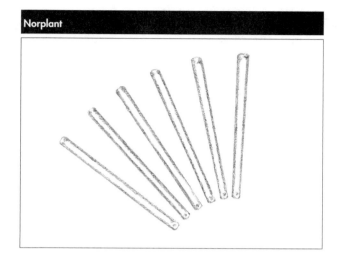

Norplant

Advantages

* can stay in for five years

* can be removed at anytime

* is always in place

* doesn't interfere with sex

* decreases blood loss and menstrual cramps during periods

Disadvantages

* *does not protect against STDs and HIV*

* is expensive

* requires minor surgery to insert and remove capsules

* may leave scarring at insertion site

* can result in no periods, or spotting or irregular bleeding

Cost

The Norplant and insertion costs $500 to $600 and removal costs from $100 to $200.

Where Can You Get It?

Norplant is currently not available in the United States, although it is available to readers in other countries.

IMPLANON

What Is It?

Implanon is a single implant inserted beneath the skin of your upper arm. It releases the etonogestrel hormone on a daily basis and is effective for three years. It prevents ovulation, thins the lining of the uterus, and thickens cervical mucus so that it stops sperm from going through the cervix.

Effectiveness

Implanon is over 99 percent effective.

Possible Side Effects

* irregular menstrual bleeding
* amenorrhea (symptom levels vary from woman to woman)

Advantages

* is simpler to insert than Norplant
* may reduce cramping or pain during periods or at the time of ovulation
* may be used by women who can't take estrogen

Disadvantages

* *does not protect against STDs and HIV*
* requires a physician for insertion and removal
* creates menstrual cycle irregularities

Cost

The cost has not yet been determined.

Where Can You Get It?

Implanon is not available in the United States, although it is available to readers in other countries. Fear of litigation may delay the introduction of new implants to the U.S. market.

ORTHO EVRA—THE "CONTRACEPTIVE PATCH"

What Is It?

Ortho Evra is ethinyl estradiol—a form of estrogen and norelgestromin—administered through a patch. The patch releases the hormones, which are absorbed directly through the skin. It operates on a twenty-eight-day cycle. You do not use the patch during the week of your period. A new patch is applied each week for three weeks in a row on the buttocks, abdomen, upper torso, or upper outer arms.

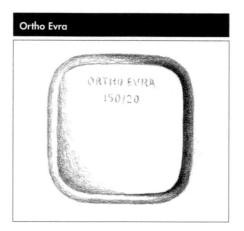

Ortho Evra

ORTHO EVRA
150/20

Effectiveness

The patch is 95 to 99 percent effective.

Possible Side Effects

✳ skin irritation

✳ allergic reaction

✳ headache

* nausea

* change in weight

* abdominal cramps

* breast tenderness

* spotty darkening of skin

* irregular vaginal bleeding

* swelling

* depression

* vaginal irritation

Advantage

* no need to think about birth control on a daily basis

Disadvantage

* *does not protect against STDs and HIV*

Cost

Otho Evra costs $30 to $35/month, plus $35 to $125 for the initial exam.

Where Can You Get It?

The patch can be administered at health centers, family planning clinics, or at a physician's office.

NUVARING

What Is It?

NuvaRing is a plastic vaginal ring containing estrogen and progesterone. It releases these hormones directly through the vaginal wall. One ring is inserted into the vagina and kept there for three weeks, then removed for one week (during menstruation), after which a new vaginal ring is inserted.

Effectiveness

The NuvaRing is 95 to 99 percent effective.

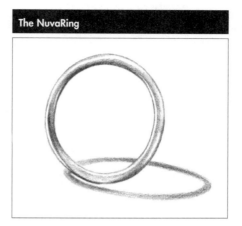

The NuvaRing

Possible Side Effects

* vaginal infection or discharge

* headache

* nausea

* abdominal cramps

* breast tenderness

* spotty darkening of skin

* rash

* weight changes

Advantages

* doesn't require daily attention

* doesn't require fitting by a clinician

* allows fertility to quickly return when use is discontinued

Disadvantages

* *does not protect against STDs and HIV*

* increases vaginal discharge

* can cause vaginal irritation or infection

Cost

The NuvaRing costs $30 to $35/month, plus $35 to $125 for the initial exam.

Where Can You Get It?

Health centers, family planning clinics, or a physician can provide the NuvaRing.

Fertility Awareness Methods (FAMs)

Fertility awareness methods (FAMs) are "natural" birth control practices that are approved by many religious groups and that are yet another way a couple can try to prevent pregnancy. FAMs require much thought and effort, and should therefore be practiced only by individuals who are willing to invest substantial energy and commitment into their birth control.

PERIODIC ABSTINENCE

What Is It?

Also called the **rhythm method, fertility awareness,** and **natural family planning,** periodic abstinence methods are based on tracking or charting your menstrual cycle in order to learn when you are fertile. Once you know this, you can avoid unprotected intercourse during those times. Charting can be done in four different ways: the calendar method, cervical mucus method, temperature method, and a combination of these methods.

Calendar method—involves calculating the time you ovulate by keeping track of your cycles for at least six months

Temperature method—requires recording daily temperature fluctuations that can indicate ovulation

Cervical mucus method—involves determining changes in vaginal mucus, which can also indicate ovulation

These methods can be combined for more effectiveness. Avoiding sexual intercourse for varying periods of time is necessary for any of these methods to work. If you choose to use any of these methods, you will need the assistance of a professional nurse practitioner or doctor to teach you how to predict your fertile period. A good book on the subject is Kass-Annese and Danzer's *Natural Birth Control Made Simple* (Hunter House, 2003).

Effectiveness

This method is typically 77 percent effective. To maximize effectiveness, it is recommended that two charting methods be used. It is not effective against STDs and HIV.

Possible Side Effects

* None.

Advantages

* is natural—no medical or hormonal side effects

* has no impact on future ability to bear children

* is acceptable to those with religious or moral concerns about birth control

* is very low cost

* is helpful when ready to become pregnant

* puts women in touch with their bodies in a unique and beneficial way

* brings couples together if they make a commitment to this method

Disadvantages

* *does not protect against STDs and HIV*

* restricts number of days allowed for intercourse

* has low efficacy

* is associated with high risk of failure unless used carefully and consistently

* requires professional instruction in observing and charting fertility signs

* is difficult to use for women with irregular menstrual cycles

* is difficult to make accurate observations due to stress, fevers, and vaginal infections

* requires daily charting of temperature and vaginal mucus

Cost

Temperature kits at drugstores cost $5 to $8 and up. Health and church centers sometimes give free classes.

Withdrawal Method

What Is It?

The withdrawal method, also known as *"coitus interruptus,"* prevents pregnancy by not allowing sperm to be released into the woman's vagina. It requires the man to take his penis out of the woman's vagina during sex *before* he ejaculates. It is probably the most ancient form of birth control and could lead to a male sexual dysfunction (premature ejaculation) if practiced enough over time. The withdrawal method is still sexual intercourse even though the man doesn't ejaculate inside the woman.

Effectiveness

Withdrawal has an effectiveness rate of 77 percent. It is *not* effective against STDs or HIV. It is not recommended for sexually inexperienced men.

Possible Side Effects

* none

Advantage

* can be used to prevent pregnancy when no other method is readily available

Disadvantages

* *does not protect against STDs and HIV*

* can cause pregnancy, since sperm can be present in pre-ejaculatory fluid

* is difficult to practice, as some men fail to withdraw completely or in time

* requires great self control, experience, and trust

* is not appropriate for men who are likely to have "premature ejaculation"

* is not appropriate for men who can't easily tell when they have to pull out

* may reduce the woman's sexual pleasure and chances of orgasm

* may reduce the intensity of the man's orgasm

Signs of Pregnancy

If something goes wrong and you're wondering if you're pregnant, look for the following pregnancy signs:

* missed period(s) or a very light, short period

* tender and swollen breasts

* needing to use the bathroom a lot

* "morning sickness"—nausea or vomiting, usually first thing in the morning

* mood and appetite changes

* discharge (wet spots) in your underwear

Note: These signs may be true for many pregnant women, but pregnancy signs differ from woman to woman. Some may have none of these signs, while others may have all of them. Furthermore, many women experience these same symptoms before they get their period. So to put your mind at rest, the best thing is to do is to take a pregnancy test! The earlier you get tested, the earlier you can begin prenatal care and/or decide if you want to carry the pregnancy to full-term.

Most home pregnancy tests look for antibodies of human chorionic gonaditropin (HCG), a hormone produced by the placenta and by the fertilized egg once it has implanted itself in the female's uterus. HCG can be detected in a pregnancy test as early as 7–10 days after conception.

While home pregnancy tests are fairly reliable when it comes to letting you know whether or not you're pregnant, it is still wise to seek out a health-care provider for testing if you think that you are pregnant.

Emergency Contraception Pills (ECPs)

WHAT IS IT?

ECPs are a brief, intense dose of ordinary birth control pills, progestin-only or combined pills with the hormones norgestrel or levonorgestrel, taken within 72 hours (three days) after unprotected sex, which can stop an unintended pregnancy. The first dose is taken *as soon as possible,* and a second dose must be taken twelve hours after the first. Popularly known as the **"morning-after" pill**, ECPs work by interrupting the process of an egg becoming fertilized and implanting itself in the uterus. They do this by creating a temporary hormone surge that disrupts the uterine lining. Using ECPs requires at least two doctor visits within forty-eight to seventy-two hours after unprotected sex. *ECPs do not cause an abortion.*

Effectiveness

ECPs reduce the risk of pregnancy by about 75 percent. If 100 women have unprotected intercourse once during the second or third week of their menstrual cycle, only 2 who use ECPs will become pregnant. The chance of you becoming pregnant in any given month, if you have unprotected intercourse in midcycle, is in the range of 25 percent to 30 percent. Therefore, the chance of pregnancy occurring if you use emergency contraception during that particular time of month decreases to less than 5 percent.

Possible Side Effects

Side effects are common, but last only a few days. About half of the women who use the pills experience nausea and about 20 percent actually vomit. Those who vomit may need to repeat a dose. Other effects are

✳ headache

✳ breast tenderness

✳ dizziness

✳ fluid retention

When Do You Use ECPs?

A women should use ECPs if

✳ she had unprotected vaginal–penile sex

✳ a condom breaks

✳ she started her pack of birth control pills a week late

✳ she has been sexually assaulted

Does Using Emergency Contraception Cause an Abortion?

Emergency contraception is *not* an abortifacient—it does not cause an abortion. It works to prevent pregnancy, not to get rid of an already established pregnancy. Medical science defines the beginning of pregnancy as the implantation of a fertilized egg in the lining of a woman's uterus. Implantation happens five to seven days after fertilization, and emergency contraceptives work *before* implantation and not after a woman is already pregnant. ECPs should be used only while under medical supervision, and a health-care provider needs to be informed of any existing conditions or other medications a woman is using. Never borrow someone else's pills!

How Are Emergency Contraceptive Pills Different from RU-486?

The French abortion pill RU-486 is a completely different drug from the birth control pills used for emergency contraception. It belongs to a class of drugs known as antiprogestins that are not yet available in the United States. RU-486 contains an antiprogesterone and synthetic steroid that help to terminate a pregnancy by interfering with the body's progesterone, a hormone that builds up the uterine lining to prepare for and maintain pregnancy. It increases contractions of the uterus, helping the body to expel the embryo. Its use as an emergency contraception is still being studied.

Cost

ECPs, plus a pregnancy test, cost about $20 to $25.

Where Can You Get It?

You will have to go to a doctor or a clinic, since ECPs require a prescription.

I hope this chapter has been helpful in informing you about the different types of contraception that are available to you (and your partner). In deciding upon a method of birth control, it is best to talk to your doctor about your needs, habits, and health condition. Your physician, a local health center or family planning clinic, or a woman in your life you trust can help you decide what's best for you.

RESOURCES

For more information on contraception, pregnancy, or abortion, call or visit the following:

National Abortion Federation Hotline: (800) 772-9100

Birth control information: www.birthcontrol.com

Condom information: www.condoms.net/?TO=/condoms/how_to_use.html

Condomania: www.condomania.com

Contraception information: (888) PREVEN2 (773-8362)

Emergency Contraception Hotline: (888) Not-2-LATE (668-2528)

National Pregnancy Hotline: (800) 311-2229

NARAL (formerly the National Abortion and Reproductive Rights Action League) on state abortion laws: www.naral.org

Planned Parenthood Federation of America: (800) 230-PLAN (230-7526) or www.plannedparenthood.org

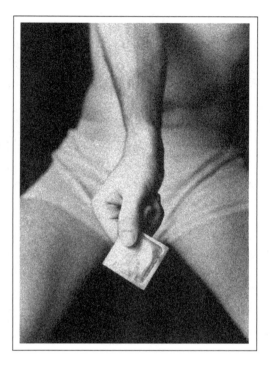

CHAPTER 9

Something to Get Sexcited About:

Safer Sex

When people start to mess around, their appetite for and infatuation with each other can quickly escalate. Before they know it, things have really progressed and that inevitable moment comes when they have to decide if it's going to be risky sex or safer sex. It's not always an easy decision. On the one hand, you should be worrying about pregnancy, STDs, and HIV and, hence, reaching for protection. But on the other hand, you're ready for some dirty, naked, animal, grunting sex, and protection is the furthest thing from your mind. While the decision to protect yourself should be quite easy, it isn't. I hope that, in reading this chapter, you'll appreciate why safer sex is the way to go, why safer sex is something to get sexcited about.

What Is Risky Sex?

Risky sex is anal or vaginal intercourse without a condom. Some people even extend that definition to oral sex without a barrier, since you might have a sore throat or small cuts on your gums (especially after you've brushed your teeth), which could make you more susceptible to STDs, including HIV.

What Is Safer Sex?

Safer sex, as defined in Chapter 1, is vaginal, anal, or oral sex practices that decrease the risk of pregnancy and of contracting STDs or HIV by reducing the amount of body fluid exchanged between partners during sexual activity.

> Less than half of U.S. college students always use condoms during sex. Almost one quarter never use condoms.

As HIV has become a greater concern among young adults, many of our peers are starting to appreciate the benefits of safer sex and to practice it. They feel that they're worth high sexual-health maintenance. Some people practice safer sex from the first time they're intimate, while for others, it comes later. It's never too late to start practicing safer sex. A number of pregnancy scares sold Cole, a 24-year-old, happenin', swingin' guy, on safer sex:

> I'm not into contraceptives like condoms, but I realize the need to use them. The emotional imbalance that comes along with not using a condom—her being more into me than I'm into her—becomes difficult to deal with. So, I think a gentleman should always wear a raincoat. I've had way too many pregnancy scares to recommend otherwise.

Practicing safer sex and making it erotic is all about your attitude and the common sense that helps you to see that protection is necessary. If you don't want to protect yourself, putting on a condom is not going to be easy or erotic. Safer sex will be a drag, and who wants that when it is unnecessary?

Practicing safer sex should come as naturally to you as putting toothpaste on your toothbrush before you brush your teeth. As long as you have a positive attitude about safer sex, then, like your pearly white, clean smile, you'll feel healthy and fresh—ready to make out and get fresh. Besides, a positive attitude will make you that much more of a sex symbol to your partner. Worrying about HIV, STDs, and pregnancy is the real damper when it comes to sex. So feel good and positive that you have control over these negative consequences by practicing safer sex. Get sexcited!!!

Nearly 80 percent of people at risk for HIV don't use condoms with a regular sex partner.

Tools for Protecting Yourself

If you have concerns about STDs, HIV, pregnancy, and potentially dishonest partners, you probably want to know more about safer sex. You may be thinking that you want to talk to your partner about it. Before you can talk about safer sex, you have to know safer-sex basics. The following four items are at the core of safer sex. Take them to heart. Use them to your advantage. They can only help to keep you and your partner healthy.

1. USE A CONDOM!!!

I can't stress enough how great these little wet suits are. Jack had his favorite brand and couldn't agree with me more: "I like Goldcoin and Lifestyles—the way they feel. They're not exceptionally thick and they grip the penis. Also, they come in cool colors. A pack of six has three different colors and the colors are a hoot!"

Note that latex condoms provide different levels of protection against different STDs. According to the Center for Disease Control (CDC), latex condoms, when used consistently and correctly, are highly effective in preventing the transmission of the following:

* HIV

* chlamydia

* gonorrhea

* trichomoniasis

Latex condoms can also reduce the risk of the following STDs:

* genital herpes

* syphilis

* HPV and HPV-associated diseases (which in turn reduces a
  woman's risk of getting cervical cancer)

One company, Condax, has gone a step further in condom promotion, researching safer sex from a perspective that challenges people's excuses for not using condoms (e.g., they're messy, smelly, interrupt the "moment," reduce sensation). Set for release in 2003, Condax Condom Applicators are specially designed plastic sleeves that are definitely a hot way to eroticize safer sex and are worth checking out:

* Kwikeze is a small, foldable plastic ring that billows, enabling a
  person to correctly install a condom on an erect penis in less
  than two seconds using only one hand.

* Zeus is a flat, bell-shaped, thin plastic device that zips the
  condom on in a flash—without interruption.

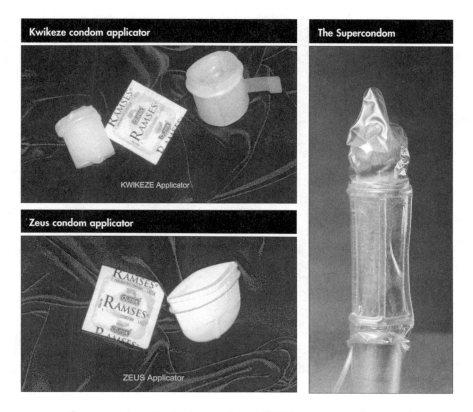

* Supercondom is the James Bond 007 license for pleasure. Not only does it automatically keep a man's penis hard (without pills, salves, or inserts), it has expandable, air-infused tubules, which are designed to hold the condom on the penis while stimulating parts of the woman's genitalia, including her clitoris.

2. DENTAL DAMS

Dental dams are latex barriers that are placed over the vagina during cunnilingus or over the anus during rimming. A lot of people aren't into them because they find them too thick for pleasure. Well, they can complain no longer. Thinner and more sensitive alternatives are available, like Saran Wrap (the nonmicrowavable kind, since the pores in the microwavable kind are bigger). Don't want to go through all the trouble of making your own dental dam? Buy some Glyde Lollyes, thinner dental dams in flavors like wild berry and vanilla. In using a dental dam, make

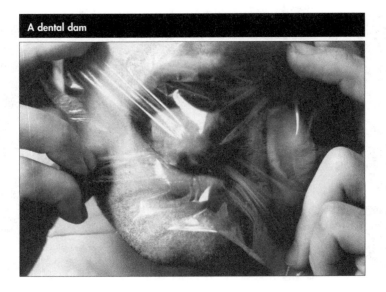

A dental dam

sure you cover the entire anus or vulva with it, holding the edges firmly with your hands. Simply stimulate the anus or vulva as you normally would. When you've had your fun, make sure to throw away the dental dam, since it should never be reused, shared, reversed, or transferred from the vagina to the anus and vice versa.

3. LUBRICANTS

To take care of the extra friction a condom sometimes causes and to help prevent breakage, use a water-based lubricant to make sex more enjoyable. K-Y Jelly is always good, but there is a whole world of latex-friendly lubricants that can be found at reputable, adult sex stores. Among them are Astroglide, Eros, ID Lube, AquaLube, or Slip for thinness, and Embrace, Probe, and Slippery Stuff Gel for thickness. For those times when you're doing it in a swimming pool or hot tub, underwater silicone-based lubes, like I-D Millennium and Wet Platinum, are also available. Lube can be tasty, too; it comes in scrumptious flavors like raspberry sorbet and champagne cocktail. Remember: Do not use oil-based lubes when practicing safer sex.

4. LATEX SURGICAL GLOVES

For those times you have a cut or sore on your hand(s) that you want to protect from possibly infected body fluids, use latex (or nonlatex polyurethane) surgical gloves. These gloves, which are available in different sizes and colors, also help to prevent the fingernails from tearing tissue during stimulation of the penis, vulva, or anus.

Talking about Safer Sex

In case you need more reasons and incentive to talk about safer sex with your partner, maybe some of the following will do the trick. You should talk to your partner about safer sex if you

* are putting your partner at risk for an STD or HIV

* want the two of you to get tested to make sure you're "clean"

* want to incorporate condoms and other forms of contraceptives or safer sex into your sex life

* are worried about STDs that show no symptoms, but can still be transmitted—you're afraid of your partner being asymptomatic, but still giving you something

* are concerned about STDs that condoms don't protect you from, like HPV

* are worried about pregnancy

A lot of couples get to a point where closeness, intimacy, and exclusivity discourage safer-sex discussions and practices. While having all of these factors in a relationship is excellent, it doesn't make the relationship risk-free. It can be hard to admit that you need to practice safer sex.

No matter how long a couple has been involved or how the relationship has developed, safer-sex discussions benefit everybody. People who are more romantically involved with their partner, who feel more loving toward their partner, and whose partner is more self-disclosing, report more extensive sexual communication anyway.

Concerns You May Have about Pregnancy, STDs, and HIV

Sometimes it can be really hard to talk about safer sex with your partner. After all, you know your lover pretty well and things should be safe and good. Or perhaps you're still getting to know each other and you don't want to spoil things with worries of pregnancy, STDs, and HIV. Who wants to come across as pushy, ignorant, or unsure and end up offending your partner or implying that the two of you have a sexual issue to work though? Talking about safer sex could be a turn-off. Plus, it could be awfully embarrassing and really distressing in a relationship to talk about sexual history and behaviors in other relationships. Certain impressions might be made. What if she thinks you have HIV? What if he thinks you've been with a lot of people? What if your partner wasn't even planning on having sex with you?!

Furthermore, part of what makes talking about safer sex difficult is that if you're a person who is not infected with an STD or HIV, you have to decide whether or not to bring up these topics at the risk of hurting your partner's feelings. Your partner could take it personally that you're suggesting that your sexual relationship may be putting you at risk.

While the embarrassment and difficulty involved in safer-sex discussions are real, don't let them stop you from protecting your health and your life. Talking about safer sex is a way of sharing responsibility and intimacy. It can help you and your partner build trust, demonstrate caring, and enable you to protect your health. Plus, sexual self-disclosure has been found to increase the sexual rewards in a relationship and overall relationship satisfaction. These, in turn, enhance sexual satisfaction. So if you want to talk to your partner, definitely do so—if not for the relationship, then for yourself. You owe it to yourself.

Frodo is one of many who realizes that he does owe it to himself:

I am a consistent condom-user just because there's always that "what if"
situation—getting pregnant, getting an STD. There's always that barrier.
There's no excuse not to use condoms, especially if you don't know
your partner. You should never be too nervous to talk to your partner.

Using protection is not an issue of not trusting your partner or what you think about them. It's just that not using it could cost you your life!

Safer sex is in vogue. Research has shown that people at high risk of getting STDs are changing their behavior—they're starting to use condoms.

HOW TO TALK TO YOUR PARTNER ABOUT SAFER SEX

In talking to your partner about safer sex, think about what you want to say, why you want to say it, and ways you can express yourself without offending your partner (though you might not be able to help this at all times). Above all, be honest. Sort out your own feelings and know the facts before you talk to your partner. It'll make things a lot easier and show that you've really thought this out. Your partner will take you and your concerns more seriously because of that.

Choose a good time to talk, one that will be free from interruptions and when the two of you won't be tired or irritable. Try to avoid this kind of talk before, during, or after sex. Your emotions are usually not under control at these times, especially if you've consumed alcohol. Pick a time when you can discuss safer sex and your relationship calmly, openly, and in a straightforward manner. Chances are that if you can handle yourself this way, your partner will be able to, too, as was the case for Veronica: "I'm stringent about using a condom every time I have sex. I don't know if my ex-boyfriend would've used one if I hadn't insisted. He respected that using a condom was important to me."

It's natural to feel uncomfortable during one of these talks, so it may help to admit that you're embarrassed and/or scared. This may also help your partner to relax and identify with you more fully. Some ways to begin a discussion on safer sex may include

✳   "I need to talk to you about something that's important to both of us. I feel a little embarrassed to be bringing this up. It's kind of hard for me, especially since I hope I'm not offending you, but I think that we really should talk about safer sex...."

* "All of this stuff I'm hearing about HIV and STDs is really scaring me. Does it scare you?... What do you think people are doing about it?... What do you think we should do about it?..."

* "Even though things have been great with us so far, I can't help but be a little worried about STDs and HIV. I've been learning about how a lot of these diseases infect the body and I just can't help but feel like we're not being safe enough when we have sex, in case we are putting each other at risk. What do you think we could do to protect ourselves?..."

After you've said your piece, give your partner time to express how he or she feels, to ask questions, and to respond to your concerns. Be prepared to hear things from your partner that may make you angry or resentful. Keep these emotions under control and prepare yourself for difficult things you may have to say. Listen carefully and ask questions if you do not understand where your partner is coming from.

In trying to resolve the safer-sex issue, move toward making it a team effort. Use the term "we" instead of "you." Own your statements by using "I" instead of projecting your thoughts onto your partner by using "you." Listen and accept what both of you have to say.

Also, when talking to your partner, make sure you make eye contact with him, nod your head when she makes a point about something, and watch your body language (i.e., have your arms at your sides instead of crossed).

INTRODUCING THE CONDOM

Regardless of where your talk goes, one of your goals is to talk about using a condom. Many people are intimidated by the idea of having to do this, but it can be as easy as saying, "Let's use a condom. I think we're worth it." Be enthusiastic and sexy when you bring up using a condom. Mention that you know of ways (and don't worry, you will after reading later chapters) to eroticize introducing a condom during foreplay. In your sexiest voice, you can say any of the following:

* "You know, wearing a condom helps me *totally* let go when we're having sex. Why don't you grab the condom I keep in my bed table drawer?"

* "Putting on a condom *really* turns me on."

* "I find men who wear condoms to be *very* attractive."

* "I've heard that using a condom makes a man last longer. Up for a sex marathon?"

* "Did you know that condom-users average three more minutes of sexual intercourse than do nonusers! I could handle three minutes more with you!"

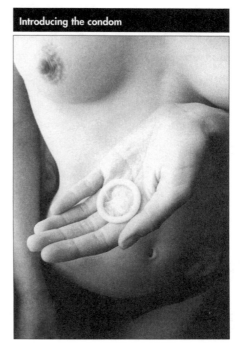

Introducing the condom

Remember, getting started is always the hardest part. Your partner may even be relieved that you're bringing up this stuff. Although these kinds of talks are serious, try to keep your sense of humor, as Madison does with her partner: "One of us will grab the protection and every now and then we'll exchange a smile as the other jokes, 'safety first.' It's pretty silly, but we're no fools."

A joke or good laugh can help both of you feel more comfortable. Also, expect to have this type of conversation more than once. As a relationship develops, different issues come up relating to safer sex. It's important to keep communicating about sexual health and protection as your relationship evolves.

One study found that 51 percent of people with two or more sex partners never use a condom with their primary partner and that 40 percent of them never use a condom with a secondary partner (the other person they're sleeping with).

I can't say enough about safer sex. Safer sex is cool! It's smart! Safer sex is about respecting yourself and your partner. Though we don't always hear our peers openly advocate for safer sex, a lot of people out there are into it and know that it's for the good of everybody, like Byron here:

> Safer sex should definitely be practiced. Just with HIV—that you can have it and not know it and be a carrier and pass it on to other people before you know you have it. Safer sex shouldn't be an issue. Even if you practice abstinence until marriage, you might want to decide when you're going to have a child. Plus, knowledge of one's partner is critical. In being intimate with somebody, you're sharing much more than a feeling.

Abstinence

We can't overlook abstinence—refraining from penile–vaginal, anal, and oral sex. Abstinence is not only a safer sex choice, but the safest choice. We are in the midst of a sexual "retro-revolution." Virginity is perceived as a more acceptable and popular choice among today's young adults, and many current virgins are proud to be in what some of my friends would call the "V-Club."

The way I see it, there are two types of abstinence out there. There's the type that people have been practicing since birth. Then there's the abstinence that is practiced by those who have opted to refrain from sexual intercourse for a period of time—"secondary abstinence." A lot can be learned from both groups in their sexual decision making. A lot can be learned, too, from how they deal with being abstinent, as Phillip, a 24-year-old, self-described recluse graduate student, shares:

> I find that limiting how often I masturbate helps me to deal with not having sex. By forcing myself to exercise some modicum of self-control, I usually restrict myself to twice per week. It gives me something to look forward to sexually. If, on the other hand, I masturbate nearly every day, I quickly become frustrated with the fact that I'm not having sex.

REASONS FOR ABSTINENCE

By the time you reached adulthood, most of you had opportunities to have sex or to consider whether you wanted the opportunity to get it on. Even though the first intercourse experience is usually unplanned, the decision to make the transition from virgin to nonvirgin is rarely spontaneous. Many people have decided to practice abstinence for a number of reasons.

For a fair number of people, about 25 percent, it is a simple matter of not having met the "right" person. For about 43 percent of virgins, it's a matter of waiting to have sex with someone they're in love with. A lot of virgins desire sex, but abstain from it because they require an appropriate reason to become sexually active.

Trey, a 24-year-old pilot, practiced abstinence for the following reasons:

> I kept my virginity for 22 years. There were three reasons I waited. First, commitment—along the lines of knowing the person, her family, the type of person she was, trusting her and confiding in her. That ties into number two—the idea of lust versus love and why I think that's important, and how that went against religious beliefs I had of what's important. And three—STDs and pregnancy. I was worried about that and wanted to keep the risk down.

SECONDARY ABSTINENCE

Even though people have been sexually active, they sometimes take a break from partner-sex. For most people, the longest they've gone without sex is over one year, with being busy or having no partner being the biggest reasons why they're not having sex. Here's why some people have abstained...

* Bernard's partner wants to wait, so he has been abstinent while dating her: "I've been abstinent for three and a half years! It wasn't easy. Isn't easy. My girlfriend now, she wants to wait 'til the big day—wedding day. We fool around, but no penetration. Masturbation is the key to living!"

* Some people, like David, a 24-year-old, outdoorsy graduate student, are just picky about a partner: "I've gone a year and two

months without sex. I haven't found anybody that I've wanted to have sex with. Consequences don't outweigh the benefits."

* Sometimes it's a dry spell, like for Nick, a 25-year-old activist: "I went for a year and a half and part of it was that I didn't date much for that year. I wasn't in a serious relationship and the couple of relationships I did have didn't progress to that."

* At times, it's a matter of taking a break from sexual relationships, as it was for Anthony, a 27-year-old, fairly conservative, graduate student: "I went a year without having sex. I'd broken up with a four-year girlfriend and wasn't ready for another relationship during that time span. I'm not really into casual sex for myself."

Plus, there's the situation of getting over heartache, as in Ashley's dry spell:

I started seeing other guys a couple of months after things ended with this guy I was crazy about. Unfortunately, none of them turned me on. For a while, it was because I was still so into my ex. Then, even though I was over him, I wasn't totally turned on to the point I'd want to sleep with any guy I was coming across. It was a year and a half before somebody finally did it for me!

If you're still wondering why safer sex is something to get sexcited about (though I hope it's clear by now!), you should know that we're going to hit on that in Part III of this book. We'll cover plenty of ways to eroticize safer sex. I wanted to address these important issues and talk to you about safer sex because we're about to have lots of protected sex in the next chapter!

RESOURCES

For more information on safer sex, call the numbers below or visit the following websites:

American Social Health Association: www.ashastd.org

Centers for Disease Control: www.cdc.gov/ or (800) 342-AIDS (342-2437)

Coalition for Positive Sexuality: www.positive.org

Planned Parenthood: www.plannedparenthood.org

The Rubber Tree, a nonprofit organization that sells interesting, safe, FDA-approved condoms: www.rubbertree.org

The Society for Human Sexuality's "Comprehensive Guide to Safer Sex": www.sexuality.org

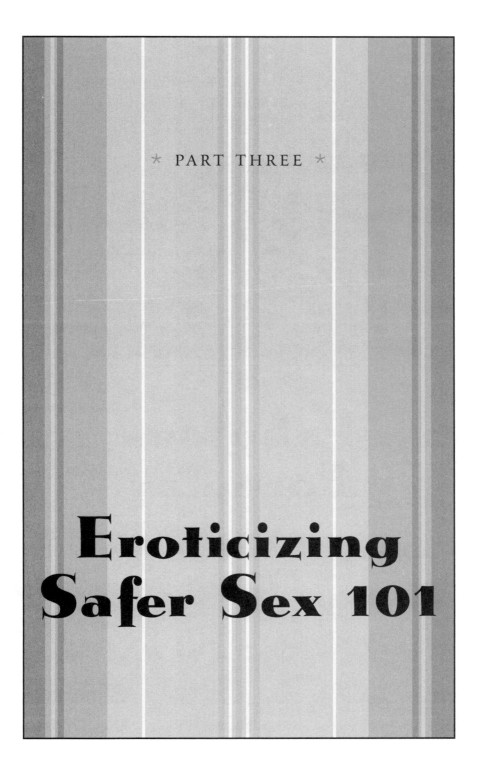

* PART THREE *

Eroticizing
Safer Sex 101

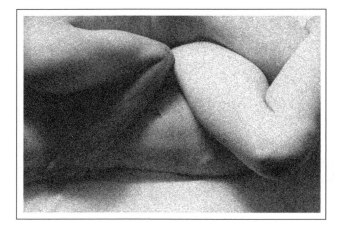

CHAPTER 10

Fabulous
Foreplay

What are some hot things you can do during foreplay?

What are some sexy ways to put on a condom?

It's that time—the pregame show. I think it'll be a star-studded foreplay performance. Sex simply isn't as stellar without it. The body feels so much better when it's warmed up and geared to go, like when you get to a hockey game before it starts. As the music blasts and the fans make their way into the stands, you stare down at the ice, watching your favorite team warm up. Your team is on its way to the Stanley Cup. There's an excitement in the air like at no other time, and your heart starts pounding, knowing that you're in for a wild time. The puck hits the ice and the game is underway and your body is gripped with excitement and anticipation. It's not too much longer now before your team is going to score!

Now think about it. How differently would you experience that hockey game without that pregame, adrenaline-pumping show? You'd feel a little cheated, right? It's fun to be involved with the match right from the start. I hate it when I walk into a sports event and the match has already started. It's the same thing with foreplay and sex. While there are definitely times when hitting the sheets without any foreplay, totally caught up in passion, can be superb, warming up simply makes for a better, bigger show.

There are as many ways to get sexy and get things underway as there are bad drivers. So many things to hit. A few don't-know-if-I-should-go-there red lights to run. A couple of rear ends to bump. I'm going to give you a few foreplay ideas that are sure to get your motors ready. Ladies and gentlemen, start your engines! Get ready to strap on a condom and go for a ride!

Pamper Your Partner

Give your partner something you probably don't give enough of—100 percent of your undivided, ardent attention. What are some good ways to do this?

* ❊ Play with your lover's erogenous zones. This could be her lips and neck, his ear lobes and chest, her breasts, his feet…. You can

try kissing them, sucking them, lightly brushing them with your fingertips, nibbling on them, stroking them....

✳   Kiss your partner. Vary your style from a sensual sucking to French kissing to hard, demanding kisses to light, teasing lip brushes. Kiss your partner all over, hitting the areas you normally wouldn't.

✳   Give a massage. Get out your body lotion or baby oil. Rub your partner all over. Don't ignore a single part!

✳   Make it your job to put on the condom before things go too far. Have your partner relax, and slip it on as you do any of the things I just listed.

Food

What better way to enjoy a snack than when it's served on your partner's body? People love to eat. People love sex. What greater love is there than combining the two? Talk about *bon appétit!* Plus, any of the edible activities that follow allow you to focus solely on your partner:

✳   Melt chocolate, like Nutella, and pour it over your partner's body, hitting some key targets. Lick it off.

✳   Take some fruit, crush it against your partner's body, then suck, lick, or eat it off.

✳   Pour some champagne over your diva and lap it up as it dribbles over her nipple, runs down her side, and drips from her mons.

✳   Make a sundae on your Playgirl and devour her, I mean it.

✳   Put something edible, like honey, on yourself. Have your partner feast on it while you put on the condom.

Pornography

Forty-seven percent of Americans have used porn to enhance sex, with 84 percent of those citizens using porn videos and 34 percent of them checking out porn magazines. Sharing in a little light erotica or hard-core porn can be just the thing you and your partner need to rev things up.

Since there's so much porn out there, I did a little investigative work for you on this one. There's lots to choose from! If you don't know much about it, how do you know when you're getting quality pornography? I didn't want to leave you totally hanging, so a few of my friends and I got together for a PPP—Pizza Porn Party—to review a few movies. The following are our top recommendations:

* *Debbie Does Dallas: The Next Generation*—As a FYI, Dallas is actually a guy. This newer version got all thumbs up at the PPP. Not only did it actually have lots of plot and dialogue, but the music was good—not that cheesy "bom chicka bom bom" that porn movies are known for. The flick also gives you tips on talking dirty, has a fantasy component, has a touch of humor, features actresses who are natural looking (no implants), and the actors practice safer sex.

* *Dangerous Tides*—You can't go wrong with the queen of pornography, Jenna Jameson. Her videos are quite the production, with lots of scenery and costuming. Jenna is one busy lady in her movies, showing you how it's done with all sorts of more-than-willing pirates, ship captains,...

* *High Heels*—This Andrew Blake film got all thumbs up as well, because it is so erotic and artistic—really quite classy compared to how cheesy a lot of porn videos can be. This all-female, aesthetically pleasing movie reminded us of a sexy R&B video, only it is more sensual, has a European flavor and setting, and is set to a nice tribal drum beat. The film's focus is actually not on sex, but everything in it is super sexy, for example, a woman shaving herself and women pouring champagne on each other.

Remember that these are videos that the PPP attendants, the majority of whom were women, found pornographically appealing. You and your partner might have completely different tastes, so find the kind of pornography that works for you. With all of the films this industry has to offer, I'm sure you'll find a handful of entertaining clips.

In some studies, women report more arousal than men when exposed to explicit materials, especially erotica involving the woman initiating sexual activity and being the focus of the activity. This could be because the plot is rather forbidden and taboo. What's ironic is that women are sometimes unaware of their physical arousal from erotica.

Strip Show

If you're feeling especially creative, energized, or seductive, put on your own striptease show. How? First, remember that timing is everything. Slowly and provocatively undress in front of your partner. If you rush, it indicates that you're not comfortable with your body or performance. So

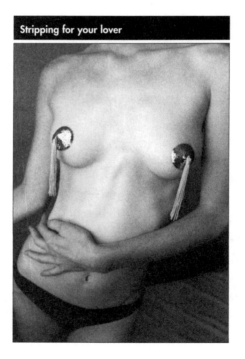

Stripping for your lover

take your time and be a visual tease. In undressing, work your way to the point where there's still a little left to the imagination.

In putting on your show, there are a bunch of things you can do. Swivel your hips. Strut around. Press yourself up against her, using a dry humping motion. Grind yourself against his body. Run your finger along your partner's lips. Brush lightly against his crotch. Stretch. Arch your back. Throw your hair back. Run your tongue over your lips. Lick yourself anywhere you feel like it. Smack your butt. Caress your neck. Suck your finger. Suck her fingers.

As you're doing all of this, make sure that you're not always making eye contact, and even turn slightly away from your partner after you've brushed up against him/her. You are a temptress. You are a rock star. You're putting on a show and your partner is your adoring fan. Give it all you've got. Oh, and don't forget that since this is just a preshow performance, you should intermittently undress your partner and put on the condom. Seeing you half-naked will keep all the sexual stamina going while you slide on his love glove.

> While I encourage men to put on such a performance for their lovers, ladies, you should definitely do this for your man at least once. Studies have found that men are more turned on by visual stimuli than women and that many of them have mild fetishes, like seeing their partners wear certain types of clothes. So get dolled up or invest in a costume, like a Catholic schoolgirl outfit. It will drive him mad!

Fantasy and Your Relationship

Because fantasy is such a personal thing, we usually equate it with solo acts. Yet while fantasies can have more of an erotic charge if kept private, when shared with a partner they can create energy you've never before seen in your sex life. Sharing sexual fantasies can add unheard-of new life and vigor to your sex life. It can also be a powerful tool in eroticizing safer sex, partly by helping to keep the relationship a monogamous one. Slipping on a condom may not always seem like the most ideal thing in the world during sex play, but think about how the whole scenario changes when you and your partner think up games, based on your fantasies, and get them rolling during foreplay!

Stuck for some ideas? Wondering what other couples are into? Among some of the most popular fantasies people have that the two of you may want to act out are the following:

* pretending you're each a member of the opposite sex

* having sex in a public place

✳ having sex with a prostitute or being a prostitute

✳ being a virgin or having sex with an inexperienced individual

✳ cross-dressing

✳ having sex with a forbidden partner, e.g., nun

✳ being in complete sexual control of your partner or being sexually owned and dominated

✳ having sex in the great outdoors

> Unspoken fantasies that you keep to yourself during sexual activity are good for sexually monogamous, long-term relationships because they introduce exciting variety, e.g., you can imagine you're with somebody else, without being unfaithful to your partner. Fantasizing is not a sign of disloyalty or dissatisfaction in a relationship!

Where's the Love?

Don't forget that expressing your feelings for your partner can be the best kind of foreplay. Whispering sweet nothings in each other's ears can allow the two of you to savor each other in a most amorous way. If he turns you on, tell him that. If she's simply irresistible, let her know. If you love each other, say it! You get the picture. Show a little soul.

Oral Fixations

One way to not only impress your partner, but also make sex erotic, is to put a condom on your partner using only your mouth. If you know how to tie a cherry stem into a knot using just your tongue, tap into that talent. You're going to be using a lot of the same action. To put a condom onto an erect penis using your mouth, do the following:

1. Unless you like the taste of spermicide, use an unlubricated, pinch-tipped condom.

2. Unroll the condom a little to loosen it up, then roll it back to its original shape.

3. Place the condom in your mouth in front of your teeth, gently holding the edges with your lips, which you've made into the shape of an "O."

4. Put your lips over the head of his penis, tighten them, push the rim over the head, and roll the condom all the way down his shaft. Use your tongue to guide it as well.

5. Make sure to run your lips up and down his penis, applying firm pressure to squeeze any air out of the condom.

6. Have your hands give it one final, snug tug to make sure it's in place.

7. And, of course, the whole time you're doing this, be a tease. You're feeling frisky! Giggle. Give him a mischievous smile. Be playful!

Note: To avoid tearing the condom, be careful not to let your teeth touch it.

CHAPTER 11

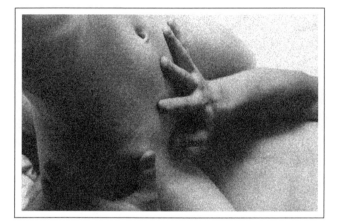

Between the Sheets and Sensational

What are some different sexual positions you could try?

What are some fabulous tips for oral sex? For hand stimulation of
the genitals?

Being a sex educator, I have had my fair share of pretty bad pick-up lines—everything from, "So if you ever need any class demonstrators, give me a ring" to "I bet that I could teach *you* a thing or two about sex." By far, the most common line has been "So what can *you* teach *me* about sex later?" Well, this chapter is about the closest thing I'll give to a private tutorial. Contained within are some rather secret and juicy tips on how to make you a more adventurous, thrill-seeking, better lover. Proceed with caution!

There are plenty of sex books out there that inform you about different sexual practices and give you the basic "how-to." What makes this chapter different is that I'm not only going to tell you how to have sex— all kinds of sex—but how to do it well. I'm a bit of a perfectionist and I wholeheartedly believe that the only job worth doing is a job done well. That's as true between the sheets as anywhere else.

Whether it's blasting, sensual, hard-core, or electric, sex is sheer physical and emotional delight, or at least it should be. Inuit Eskimos of the Arctic region call sex "laughing time," and if you're with the right love, doing the right thing, with just the right touch, it can be that good of a time. Someone once said, "Sex is the most fun you can have without smiling." While I'm sure that's true for some people, some of the time, it's certainly not the rule.

Sex can sooo make you smile. Sex can make you laugh. Sex is a romp that brings out the kid in you. Sex is a chance for your body to play and feel and touch as it can in no other way. Sex can bring you closer to someone you care about, helping you better understand and appreciate your partner. Sex is a way of expressing your love for somebody. Sex is something you and your lover can really get into, actively and passionately creating your own altered state of mind.

Sensational sex is a constant exchange of energy and rapture, as Jordan, a 25-year-old student with the nicest, whitest smile, describes: "Sex is a two-way street. I enjoy sex more when it's going back and forth between my girlfriend and me, like when you're with a friend on a roller coaster and both of you are having fun. We're doing something together and not having sex just for having sex.... You're doing something you both like to do."

Sex should make you feel so wonderful that nothing in this world can wipe that big ol' smile off your face as you come down from it. It should be that fabulous!

> Good sex doesn't just happen naturally. It takes a lot of work on the part of both part-ners. Furthermore, the best kind of sex involves intimacy, and intimate sex is a learned ability. Intimate sex is more than just making love. It is the process of enhancing the love you feel for your partner, sharing it, and celebrating it.

SexSexSex

The room is charged with a fiery fervor. All you want now is to feel his pulsating penis in you, hear her gasp as you first enter her, and for the two of you to go at it like you never have before. I'm sooo with you here, but before you go any further, if you haven't already, whip out that condom!

Intercourse Positions

MISSIONARY

Also known as the "**Man on Top**" position, the woman is on her back and the man is on top of her, between her legs. This position gives the man a great deal of control and movement, while the woman's movements are limited. Most men like this position because it provides for excellent access to all of his partner's body parts and it gives him control over thrusting—namely the intensity and depth of it. This position fulfills the male need to be dominating and wanted by his partner.

Most women like the missionary because it meets their romantic needs of wanting to be taken care of and/or dominated. The woman is easily stroked by her partner, and she doesn't have to do a lot of work. This posi-tion is nice in that it allows the couple to look into each other's eyes, kiss, and note each other's full reactions as they communicate their love, lust, and desires.

Another way this position can be enjoyed is for the woman to bring her legs up and wrap them around her partner's back, thus increasing genital contact for both partners. This gives her more control of the angle and the depth of his thrusts, and to spice things up, she can become a black widow spider, squeezing her lock around him tighter and tighter as things become more carnal. This position also causes the woman's pelvis to tilt so that she experiences more sensations.

FEET ON SHOULDERS

In this position, the woman is on her back and can either bend her legs back onto her chest or stretch her legs back by her ears. The man enters her from on top. This position allows for great deep penetration and, as a result, *queefing,* a vaginal "fart," may occur. Remember that sex is "laughing time," so just laugh if this happens.

WOMAN ON TOP

The simplest way to get into this position is for the woman to lie on top of her partner with her legs outside of his. This is most easily done from a side-embrace, during which she'll swing her leg over the side of his body, climb onto him, and lower herself onto his erect penis.

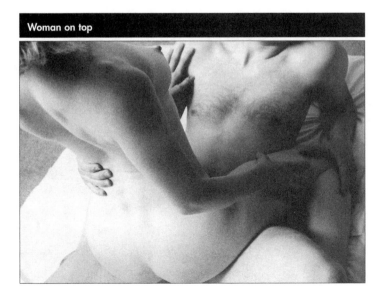

Woman on top

"I like it on top. I have more control—not that I'm a control freak, but it gives me more control of what feels good," says Veronica, and she speaks for many females on this one. This position is so popular among women because it allows for direct stimulation of the clitoris during intercourse. Not only can a woman enjoy playing horsey for a little while, but she can also control the depth of penetration and the speed and angle of the man's thrust when she's on top. A major advantage of this position is that a man can caress her clitoris with his fingers as she rides him. He can also rub her breasts with his hands and touch other parts of her body during sex.

Men also make out well with this position. This position allows for more blood flow to his pelvic erectile tissue, making his penis more sensitive to stimulation. She can also do more work for her man, by moving up and down and by controlling the depth of penetration. The guy can also get excited by watching her vagina ride him and by playing with her breasts, which are in full view if she is sitting up. Plus, knowing that his partner is in more control of her own stimulation, a guy can concentrate on his own kicks and arousal.

This position has several variations. A woman can bring her legs inside the man's, allowing for a snugger genital fit and more friction between the vagina and pelvis. Or a woman can slowly lift herself upright so that she's sitting on top of her partner, placing most of her weight on her knees. This

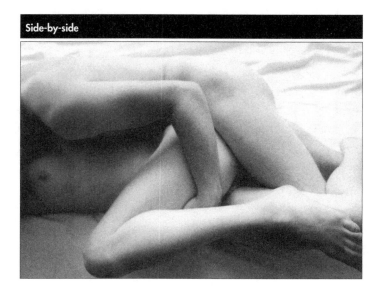
Side-by-side

position can be altered slightly as well, with the female leaning back onto his thighs.

SIDE-BY-SIDE

Both partners lie on their sides and face the same direction. The man enters the woman, who has drawn her knees upward, from behind. With her legs drawn upward, this position offers the woman deep penetration. She and/or her partner can have crazy fun playing with her clitoris if she leans back onto her partner. This is a great position if you want to take your time, be comfortable, and stay relaxed, plus this position allows for a great deal of body contact and caressing.

DOGGIE-STYLE/REAR-ENTRY

Usually the woman is on all fours and the man is on his knees and enters her from behind. This position allows the man to thrust deeply, to angle his penile movements, and to aim for his partner's G-spot. All of this gives him a great sense of dominance, which he totally gets off on. Variations of this

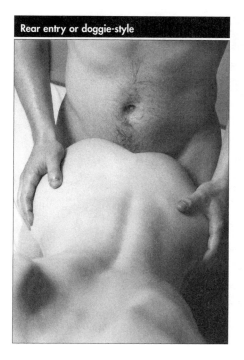

Rear entry or doggie-style

position include the woman lying on her stomach, with her back arched, so that her rear end is in the air. If she lies completely flat and squeezes her legs together, then her clitoris and labia minora are stimulated during thrusting.

STANDING

Both partners are standing upright in this position. The man can either enter the woman from the front or from behind. The woman should lift one of her legs and turn it outward so her partner can slide in before he slightly lifts her off of the ground. When entering her from the front, if the man is strong enough, he can hold the woman if she wraps her legs around

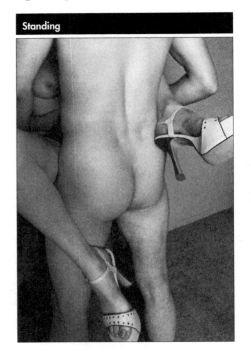

Standing

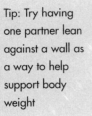

Tip: Try having one partner lean against a wall as a way to help support body weight

him. Her arms should also wrap around his shoulders so that she can better support herself and she should press her thighs against his hips for greater support. This position is easier to do if the partners are the same size, and can be quite tiring.

SITTING

This is a very intimate position that, unfortunately, gives very little genital stimulation. The man is in a sitting position and his partner straddles him. She can draw herself up against his body and move up and down on him,

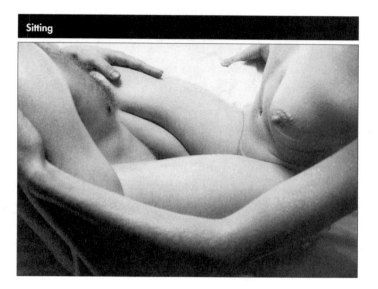

Sitting

or they can both lean back, with one taking the lead in the penetration motion. This position can also take place while sitting on a chair and can allow the woman to face her partner, sit on top of him sideways, or face away from him.

Other Sexual Behaviors

Sexual intercourse (**coitus**) is usually considered the ultimate in sexual activities between people who have reached a certain level of intimacy, whether that be in five minutes or five years. Often, couples get into a routine when it comes to having sex, forgetting that we have a wide array of sexual behaviors to choose from when we are sexually active. In maintaining monogamy, practicing abstinence, and eroticizing safer sex, people may want to consider sexual behaviors other than penile–vaginal intercourse. Some of these sex acts make for great foreplay, too.

ANAL SEX

Bottoms up! Anal–penile intercourse is a behavior that, depending on which study you look at, 10 to 40 percent of heterosexual women and 20 to 30 percent of heterosexual men have participated in. While some couples find anal sex disgusting and immoral, having an "exit-only" attitude about the anus, other couples love it, saying that it feels good, provides a tighter feel than the vagina, and is great for prostate stimulation. When you consider that the anus and rectum are full of sensitive, responsive nerve endings, plus that the G-spot, perineum, prostate gland, and the bulb of the male's penis can be stimulated during anal sex, it is no surprise that many couples enjoy anal sex. Furthermore, the rush of doing what our culture has deemed forbidden territory can be enough joy in itself.

Anal sex is somewhat more difficult than coitus because the rectum has no natural lubrication and because it's surrounded by fairly tight muscles. It is typically done with both partners face down in a rear-entry position or in a man-on-top position. Couples often opt for anal sex when the woman has an extremely heavy menstrual flow, or for variety, or simply because they want to explore the pleasures the rectum has to offer, or because the anus sometimes provides more stimulation and tightness than an overly slack vagina.

For some individuals, the anus is the most erogenous zone on their body and, for even more people, anal sex gives a deep feeling of sexual pleasure that is unobtainable in other ways. Some women report orgasm during anal intercourse, especially when accompanied by hand stimulation of the clitoris. Gay men also report orgasm during anal intercourse, primarily due to stimulation of the prostate—something any heterosexual guy can experience as well, depending on the kind of sex toys he and his partner are into.

Some people would rather not have anything to do with anal sex. This could be because they consider it to be a gay male behavior and their homophobia kicks in, or they're afraid of possible pain and tearing, or they think that it's dirty. (If cleanliness is what's holding you back, you should know that normally there's only a small amount of fecal matter in the anal canal or rectum.) Other people have the very valid concerns of the risk of HIV transmission that is tied to anal sex and of the condition of *inconti-*

nence, the loss of your anal sphincter muscle tone, that can result if the act is performed too often over a long period of time.

Haywood Jay, a 28-year-old bartender, feels that he could only ever have anal sex if it was with a one-night stand: "Anal sex—it's dirty. Taboo. So I would have trouble doing it with a partner. But with a one-night stand, I'd want to see how far she'd go. The thought's a turn on. But I'm not really into it."

Many individuals have braved the uncharted territory of the anus to find that it is a source of amazing pleasure. John Boy, a 24-year-old computer programmer/part-time masturbation specialist, describes his anal ventures:

> To me, discovering anal sex with my girlfriend was like sifting through the cobwebs in the basement to find a forgotten treasure. Society has convinced us that the anus is a dirty place, but it has far less exposure to germs than any other external areas of the body. In order to discover it, you have to rid yourself of these feelings. If you are convinced that the anus is dirty, then you are going to be tense during anal play. Tension in this area causes pain and discomfort.

> I feel the nerves in this area are more sensitive than the nerves anywhere else on my body. So just relax and enjoy! Have I received pleasure from my anus? At least once a week. How? From my fingers during masturbation to other's fingers during foreplay to dildo and butt plugs, the pleasure I receive from my anus is limitless and exquisite.

> Some of the greatest moments in my life have been achieved while orgasming during a hand job with a finger in my anus massaging my prostate.

Anal Sex "How-To"

You'll first need a few key ingredients for a successful and pleasurable anal sex venture: desire, relaxation, trust, communication with your partner, and *lots* of lube. If you have all of these, anal sex should be a pain-free, arousing, and, maybe even orgasmic experience for you and your partner. Oh, and another thing: As with any other kind of sex, make sure you have a bowel movement before you have anal sex. It'll make things much more comfortable.

Begin by moistening your partner's anus with saliva or lubricant (not Vaseline!). PrePair is a spermicidal lubricant that can be used along with condoms for anal intercourse. Lubricate the condom, and gently insert the condom-covered penis into the rectum. If the receiving partner is not relaxed enough for insertion, try relaxing the anal sphincter muscle with some finger penetration first. Another option is having the receiving partner in the "on top" position, where the penis can slide in perhaps a tad more easily, allowing the receiver to have more control.

No matter which position you choose, throughout an anal sex experience, try to maintain a controlled pelvic thrusting so that you can take care not to tear either the anal lining or the condom. Doing things slowly, especially at first, is key to making anal sex work for you and your partner. Make sure you check in with your partner regularly, too, to make sure that your lover is comfortable and not in pain.

If you're the recipient, *relax.* The more you can relax, the more comfortable anal sex will be. Know that if it is done properly, anal sex does not need to involve pain. In following this advice, perhaps you can have a better first-time anal sex experience than Shirl-dog did: "I only tried anal sex once and it was so difficult. The girl didn't like it. The main pleasure I got from it was trying to do it and getting it done. I was turned off from doing it again."

Many couples may want to experiment with anal sex. As long as both partners are cool with it, there's no harm in experimenting with it, using lots of lubrication and a condom. The lubrication will prevent condom breakage and the condom may end up saving your life, protecting you from HIV and other STDs.

Tip: Never insert a penis (or your fingers or a sex toy) into the vagina after anal sex unless a new condom is being used or the penis (or fingers or toy) has been washed thoroughly. Bacteria from the rectum can cause vaginitis if introduced to the vaginal canal.

ANALINGUS

Analingus is the tongue and mouth stimulation of the anus, a.k.a. "rimming," or "tossed salad," which 36 percent of men and 39 percent of women are into. In performing analingus, make sure that you use a barrier method, like a dental dam or nonmicrowavable Saran Wrap, over your partner's rectum to decrease your chances of contracting an STD or other infection. By not using a barrier, you are placing yourself at a greater risk for acquiring hepatitis B or E-coli infections.

Analingus "How-To"

To perform analingus on your partner, begin by playing with the buttocks and perineum, kissing and licking the area. Slowly work your way to your partner's rectum. Lick the perimeter of the anus in an up/down motion, or try circling it, pointing your tongue while practicing a flicking motion. Try probing the inside of the anus a bit, darting your tongue in there every now and then. Nibble. Suck. Remember, using a dental dam of some sort is going to help you relax more, easing you of cleanliness and STD concerns.

GLUTEAL SEX

Gluteal sex, while it sounds really different and exotic, is a fairly simple and super alternative for couples who don't want to have anal sex, but who want to experience some of the same mental and physical pleasures of anal sex. During gluteal sex, the man uses the crease of the woman's buttocks when he thrusts. As the woman contracts her gluteal muscles and rotates her pelvis, the man can thrust into the crease. Because there's going to be lots of skin-on-skin during this kind of sexual activity, it's still a brilliant idea to use a condom for whatever protection it can offer against STDs. Lubrication is also going to help, since the crease won't provide you with any natural lubrication and things could get quite sore without it.

ORAL SEX

Oral sex is a standard sex technique that about three-quarters of the U.S. population engages in, with most of those people loving it. Some of the most enthusiastic cunnilingus lovers are men ages 25 to 29, with almost half of them saying they like oral sex "very much." Of the men and women not crazy about the act, many cite smell, taste, seeing genitalia, performance anxiety, and discomfort as reasons they're not into oral sex.

PLO-Style, a 22-year-old fly kind of guy, gives his take on oral sex:

I'm not big on receiving it. I like it, but would rather give it. When guys go out, they're like "I wanna get my dick sucked," whereas I'm like, "I wanna lick some pussy." I like it when a girl climaxes. It turns me on so much. I just like having my face down there. I'm the president, founder, and leader of the P.L.O.—the Pussy Licking Organization (laughs). I love how a woman reacts to it.

There are lots of reasons why oral sex has become so popular in recent years. With more young people concerned about HIV and STDs, people are realizing that oral sex is a sumptuous way to lower their risk of HIV and STD transmission, especially with the use of a dental dam or condom, while still being sexually active. I have to note here, however, that while the risk of HIV and STD transmission during oral sex is lower than vaginal–penile and anal intercourse, its risk of transmission is higher than was originally thought.

Benefits of Oral Sex

* feels amazing

* no risk of pregnancy

* super form of foreplay

* can be a substitute for intercourse

* adds variation to sexual activity

* orgasm can happen quickly and intensely because sexual pleasuring is so concentrated

Cunnilingus

"Going down" on a girl, "eating her out," "muff munching"—it's all about stimulating a female's genitals with your mouth. *Cunnilingus* literally translated from Latin means "to lick the vulva." For some women, it is the best way, or only way, to have an orgasm.

This technique is becoming more and more popular among young, educated people. It is often viewed as an act that signals sexual proficiency. In addition to women finding it spectacular, most men, like Haywood Jay, adore it: "I love it. Absolutely love it! I get so erotically aroused performing oral sex on a woman. I've achieved orgasm while giving oral sex from the arousal of having stimulated a woman. It turns me on that much. When I do it, I give it 100 percent of my attention and use lots of spit!"

Cunnilingus "How-To"

Since the female genitals are such an intricate work of art, the possibilities for how to perform cunnilingus are almost infinite. Start by kissing her inner thighs and working your way to her treasure. Focus on her clitoris, using your tongue to stimulate it and the surrounding area with a quick darting and/or thrusting movement. Or you could simply press your lips around her clitoris and suck on it, or take it between your lips and lick it intensely.

Because focusing on the clitoris can get pretty intense for her, ease off every now and then, and suck on her inner lips. Or you can use your tongue to stimulate the vaginal entrance with licking motions, or even stiffen and harden your tongue and insert it into her vagina.

Once you have her begging for you to go back to her clitoris again, gradually work your way from her vaginal lips to her clitoris and move your tongue from side to side across it—slowly at first, then moving at a more rapid speed. You can also move your tongue upward from the entrance of the vagina to the clitoris and then across the clitoris. Vary keeping your tongue soft and gently caressing her clitoris, and tightening your tongue to somewhat of a point and rhythmically licking her. Feel free to use wide, sweeping strokes or to completely zero in on the clitoris.

The insertion of one or two fingers into the vagina or anus while you're doing this, or sucking on her clitoris at the same time, often produces high stimulation for the woman, sending her over the edge in many cases.

Remington, a 21-year-old student, sheepishly smiles as he remembers all of the times he's gone down on a girl using such techniques during cunnilingus:

> I absolutely love it! It's a fantastic sex act, kind of a reverse power-type thing. I'm serving somebody else's needs as opposed to having my own met. I like it all right in my face . . . the smells, her juices—though depending on the time of month and day, it can be a turn-off. But the smell . . . it's a scent you can only smell on a woman. . . . For variety, I'll occasionally use an ice cube, and I definitely have to work the fingers in.

Her clit's important. I alternate between using my tongue and fingers on it or sometimes use them at the same time, with my finger up her vagina or anus, too. I base my performance and how long to do it on if the girl's into it and her hips start grinding, and when she starts breathing deep and squeezes my head with her legs. It's best when she really shows she likes what you're doing.

If you want her panting like she's in heat the next time you go down on her, the following should do the trick. A good prelude to going down on a girl is kissing and fondling her inner thighs or belly, and then kissing the outside of her vaginal lips, arriving at the point where you can put your tongue inside the inner vaginal lips and move it in various ways. Note that it's best to start with "less" when performing oral sex, especially if you're not sure what your partner enjoys. Every woman is different and starting out "too rough" or "too fast" could really turn her off to oral sex. Plus, starting out *really* slowly is sooo tantalizing and excites your lover even more.

Have her help you out by telling you what feels good for her at that moment. Know that what is highly satisfying one minute for a woman can be painful the next, what is too fast at the beginning may be too slow toward climax, and what is satisfactory one night may be unsatisfactory the next.

Note: Come up for air every now and then!

Cunnilingus Tips

✳   Insert a finger into the vagina or anus for added stimulation. (Don't use the same fingers in the anus as in the vagina!) Some women really like this. Make sure, though, that you don't do this right away. Build up to this!

✳   Hold the labia apart to further explore her clitoris for more direct stimulation—if she can handle it.

✳   Once you've found a spot that has her screaming like a banshee, keep up your tongue rhythm in that area.

✳   Suck on a menthol or mint cough drop before you go down on her so that the sensation feels cool and tingly—refreshing. Ahhhh.... If you want to place the cough drop inside her vagina, suck on it for a while to make sure that the cough drop is round and smooth and slide it in with your tongue.

✳ With a smooth ice cube melting in your mouth, go down on her. Or use the ice to keep your fingers or tongue cool so that she can feel the different temperatures when you lick and touch her. You can even work the ice inside her with your tongue or fingers.

✳ Drink some hot coffee, tea, or water so she can feel a really warm tongue against her vulva. You can even switch back and forth between cooling your tongue with ice, then warming it with the warm drink to drive her crazy.

✳ Make a little bit of noise. You're hungry and your appetite for her is insatiable! Let her know!

✳ Don't forget about the rest of her body, especially her breasts!

✳ Use your hands to stimulate other parts of her body while you're getting her off, and/or use sex toys to enhance this sex session.

✳ Even if you're not into going down on her, act like you are. Moan, smile, challenge yourself to get into it—put on a show. (Note: If you aren't really into this, don't do it. Sex should be fun for everybody involved and if oral sex turns you off, then you and your partner can find lots of other things you both love.)

Fellatio

Fellatio, the stimulation of the penis with the mouth, is from the Latin word *fellare,* meaning "to suck." It is an in-and-out motion of moving the lips down toward the base of the penis and then back up. Since the mouth's inner lining is similar to that of the vaginal walls, fellatio produces many of the same pleasures vaginal sex does, only sometimes with greater stimulation and grip than sexual intercourse.

Fellatio "How-To"

Take his penis into your mouth and start sucking. You can change from the in-and-out motion that imitates the thrusting of the penis in the vagina, to moving your tongue in a circular fashion around the top of the penis.

Whatever your sucking rhythm and motion, begin gently at first, and then more rapidly. For variety, you can flick your tongue horizontally across the corona of his penis as well. You can also move from the penis to the testicles from time to time, taking them or a portion of them into your mouth, sucking gently. Or you can combine any of these movements. You'll have him whimpering in no time.

Note: Fellatio should consist mainly of up-and-down movements rather than sucking.

To get the guy to come, focus on the in-and-out movement, with the penis going deeper and deeper into your mouth, faster and faster. You can keep your hand loosely encircling the base of his penis and move your hand and mouth rhythmically up and down the shaft, with the hand acting in a sort of "milking" fashion as it tightens around the penis.

When performing fellatio, take your time—touching and kissing his other erogenous zones too. Men can get very impatient during oral sex, anticipating the moment of climax, so have fun dragging it out. Torture him for a little while. He will be putty in your hands. I guarantee it.

> **Men:** Some women detest it when a male places his hands on her head in order to control her motion. Don't do this unless you've asked her if she's cool with it. Let her have control of her movements. You can coach her, and even rest your hands on her head, but don't control her head by moving it or thrusting her mouth unless she's okay with it.

Fellatio Tips

✳ Cover your teeth with your lips and move your mouth up and down without grazing your teeth against his manhood. Contact with sharp teeth is a no-no.

✳ If your partner is uncircumsized, make sure not to cause discomfort by pulling the foreskin back too far.

✳ Tighten your lips as you move up and down his shaft.

✳ Lick and suck at the same time.

✳ Put a few drops of a breath mint on your tongue and blow on his penis, or rub some of the mint on his penis and then blow.

✳ "Tea bag" him for a while—that is, concentrate on just sucking gently on his testicles.

✳ Have a shot of schnapps, then go down on him. This has an effect similar to the mints.

✳ Hum while you're at it!

✳ Use scented massage oil, as Veronica has done: "Using a Victoria's Secret massage oil with my boyfriend was cool. It made my skin against his sooo smooth. It had a vanilla scent and all I could think of was *Cosmo* saying, "Lick it like an ice cream cone.""

✳ Give him head through his pants sometime if he's wearing a lightweight fabric. Seeing his trousers all wet can excite him terrifically, and the act makes for a little variety.

✳ Even if you're not totally into giving head, act excited. When you can, seductively smile at him and give him happy faces, and make noises—you know, some "ummm's"—like it's really yummy and you're *loving* it! (Note: If you aren't really into this, don't do it. Sex should be fun for everybody involved and if oral sex turns you off, then you and your partner can find lots of other things you both love.)

Gagging while Giving Head

I know that there are women who aren't crazy about giving head. The gag reflex can kick in, making a lady feel a little bit sick and yucky. The way to deal with that gag reflex is to hold his penis steady and relax your throat muscles while keeping the front part of your mouth firm enough to provide stimulation to the penis—really concentrate on this. Breathing through your nose helps. If you're able to do this, while firming your lips around his shaft to provide more stimulation to the penis, you are his sex goddess.

To Spit or to Swallow?

That is the question. About 18 percent of females spit while performing oral sex, while 41 percent swallow the semen. Most of these 41 percent will also swallow only if they're in a steady relationship. The rest stimulate the penis with their hand after sucking on it, avoiding the last-minute decision entirely. This is a pretty smart tactic since having a guy unload one in your mouth can put you at risk for STDs and HIV. Using a condom during oral sex is the best way to avoid anything being transmitted and to avoid the spit or swallow last-minute decision.

For those of you who have never swallowed, you're not missing much. The ejaculated semen gives a sensation of warmth in your mouth. The semen has little taste at first, but later becomes salty. Some men prefer that their partner swallow the semen, saying that it feels better and is more intimate—that it's a positive sign if she does so. While it's a nice gesture, it's your body and your health and it's just as loving of him not to insist that you swallow it. It's your call—your life. If you choose to swallow his cum, though, for whatever the reason, and don't want to taste the semen, swallow quickly.

"69" (SOIXANTE-NEUF)

During "69" sex play, partners perform oral sex on each other at the same time. This can be done either with both partners side-to-side or with one person on top, lying the opposite direction of the person on the bottom. No matter what the positioning, the goal is to end up with your partner's genitals in your mouth. Game on.

Buck, a 20-year-old student, loved doing 69 with his ex-girlfriend:

> She'd be doing her thing. I'd be doing my thing. Then she'd stop because she was coming. If I told her to keep going, she would go crazy to the point it would hurt because she'd be sucking and squeezing me too hard. I didn't orgasm, but her going nuts told me that I was getting her off. Afterwards, we'd have sex and sex would always be so much better. Sixty-nine is an awesome prelude to the sexual encounter on the horizon.

This position can be great because both partners can enjoy sexual stimulation at the same time—the feeling of total body involvement. Yet, some people do not like sixty-nining because it may feel more complicated than enjoyable—too much is going on all at once. It's hard to take it all in, to give and get pleasure at the same time can be quite overwhelming and a lot of work. Taking turns sucking, while in position, can help take care of this problem.

For a lot of women who find themselves on the bottom during 69, the experience can be even less enjoyable since they may feel like they have no control over their movements or may feel like they're being choked. So, if this is the case, make sure she's on top. Sixty-nining, however, is definitely an activity worth trying at least once!

Masturbating Each Other

Masturbating each other is a great way of showing your lover what turns you on, what feels good. Mutual masturbation can be the best way for the two of you to get to know the other's body better. Whether you take turns masturbating each other or masturbate each other at the same time, such sex play can also help you get more connected and give you more control over achieving simultaneous orgasm, if that's what you desire.

Sven highly recommends this sexual activity: "Mutual masturbation is really exciting, extremely actually, in a way that pleasuring each other through sex wouldn't be. In the process of it, you're showing each other how you like to be touched. You're like, 'I can make myself feel this good. Can you make me feel this good?' "

> If you have any open cuts or sores on your hands or fingers, it's an especially good idea to use latex gloves while manually stimulating your partner, to prevent the transmission of HIV.

STIMULATING HIS PENIS WITH YOUR HAND— A "HAND JOB"

The first thing you want to do is get him erect. You can do this by rolling the penis, like dough, between the palms of your hands. Another way to make him erect is to apply firm pressure with one finger midway between the base of his penis and the anus. Once again, I'm going to point out that lube may be the perfect aid to getting the job done, and done well at that.

Once erect, the best place to grip him is right below the groove of his glans. If he's uncircumcised, avoid rubbing his glans and pull his foreskin back as far as it will go. Take one of your hands and press hard near the root, holding his penis steady or fondling his scrotum. With your other, make the thumb and first finger into a ring or use the whole hand to grip his shaft. You can vary your hand movements, and if you plan to be doing this for a while, have your hands take turns with what they're doing so you don't get tired. No matter what, it's the motion—the rhythm—of your stimulation, with just the right amount of pressure, that gets him off more than anything.

Have him show you what he likes if you get tired at any point or are wondering if there's something he wishes you were doing. One trick, if you're tired or want to further excite him, is to start playing with yourself while you get him off.

OTHER MALE-GENITAL-STIMULATION TECHNIQUES

* Once his penis is erect, cup his balls with one hand. With the heel of your other palm, glide all the way up and down the underside of the penis.

* Take the penis in one hand and for ten seconds sensuously, gently caress it before giving it one quick up-and-down stroke. Repeat, caressing his penis with slow up-and-down strokes for another ten seconds, and then give the penis two quick up-and-down strokes. Repeat the caressing, then give three quick strokes and continue this process, each time increasing the number of quick strokes until he orgasms!

* Hold the penis in one hand and with the well-oiled or lubed palm of the other hand, slowly massage the head of his penis, reversing directions every now and then.

* Place your hands on either side of his penis. Now push hard against his manhood and lift your hands up and down.

* Alternate your hands in an upward "milking" motion. Start at the base of the penis and work your way up past the tip. You can perform this motion "backwards," moving downward as well.

* Slowly and lightly run a finger up the underside of his penis. Have him tell you where the most sensitive spots are. Then squeeze, pinch, nibble, and tease it.

For techniques involving one hand, put your other hand to use. Here are some suggestions for that idle hand:

* Tease his nipples or other favorite erogenous zones.

* Massage his chest or legs.

* With a lubricated or oiled hand, rub his perineum or anus.

* Tickle or cup his testicles.

* Gently tug on the hairs covering his testicles.

* Wrap your thumb and index finger either around the penis between the balls and the body or the testicles and the shaft. In contracting slightly, your hand becomes a live cock ring.

* Lightly scratch his scrotum with your fingernails.

* Caress his penis between your breasts.

Take your partner's hand and put it over yours while you're masturbating yourself. By feeling the tempo and pressure you use, your partner can learn to use the same technique on you. Then you don't have to do all of the work! Plus, it's so erotic!

STIMULATING HER GENITALS WITH YOUR HAND

You may be getting sick of hearing me say this by now, but have some lube handy in case you need it. Begin with gentle, light strokes on the inside of her thighs and her inner and outer lips, moving to a light stroking of the clitoris. With increased arousal, stimulation of the clitoris can become firmer. You can move a couple of your fingers across her clitoris in circular or back and forth movements. Use vibrating motions, rapidly brushing your fingers across the clitoris.

Her inner and outer vaginal lips can also be stroked, rubbed, or tugged. Furthermore, you can place the heel of your hand on the mons, exerting pressure on it while moving your middle finger in and out of the vaginal entrance. Pressing against the front wall of the vagina while doing this will help her reach orgasm.

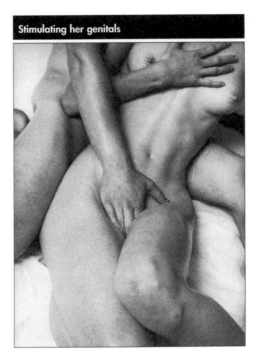

Stimulating her genitals

SOME RULES TO KEEP IN MIND WHEN MASTURBATING HER

✳ Make sure your nails are closely trimmed and do not have any jagged edges.

✳ The clitoris is sensitive—stimulation can be exquisite or painful, so make sure her reactions are from pleasure and not pain.

✳ Never rub her clitoris dry. Use a lube, saliva, or her vaginal lubrication to make stimulation of the clitoris more comfortable and luscious.

✳ For some females, direct stimulation of the clitoris is painful in some states of arousal. If this is the case with your partner, try rubbing the sides of her clitoris and inner lips instead.

✳ No matter what you're stimulating, keep up the rhythm.

OTHER IDEAS FOR STIMULATING HER

* With your well-oiled or lubed hand over her labia, fingers pointing toward her anus, pull up toward her stomach. Repeat a few times and vary the rhythm. Take the time to explore and pull at her inner and outer lips with your fingers. Take turns rubbing each gently between your thumb and forefinger.

* Insert your first two fingers into her vagina and arch your thumb back, as if hitchhiking, until it finds her clitoris. By thrusting, twisting, and vibrating your hand and fingers, you can hit both her clit and G-spot.

* Find out what her favorite spots are and lick and caress the area right around the spot, but only target in on her favorite areas every now and then. Such teasing is likely to postpone her orgasm and make it much stronger and more powerful when she finally does come!

* Insert a couple of fingers into her vagina. Take your thumb and place it against her anus, without inserting it. While you stimulate her with your fingers, apply pressure with your thumb.

* Lightly, just tickle the clitoris.

* Try asking her what she enjoys. She'll be able to tell you!

* Kiss and touch her all over.

One survey found that 35 percent of people have masturbated while another person has watched. It's yet another way to turn yourself into a real-live *Penthouse* Pet or Maverick while keeping sex play safe and erotic!

Interfemoral Sex

This is total skin-on-skin stimulation, which is why it's once again wise to use a condom for whatever protection it provides against STDs. No intercourse takes place. Instead, the man moves his penis between the thighs of his partner. The partner can squeeze the legs together, varying the amount of pressure on his tool.

Afterplay

You've just had quite the sexual encounter and are starting to realize that the rest of the world still exists. You're back on earth and are ready to...crash. But wait!

This is the time for afterplay, and afterplay can be your trump card. This is where you totally win your lover over, and once and for all prove that you're *the* best lover that has ever existed. This is also a time where if you don't play that card and if you withdraw completely, you can leave your partner hanging and wondering if everything you did wasn't really all that. So here are some afterplay pointers:

*   Don't complain about anything, especially about the sex you just had.

*   Don't jump out of bed to clean yourself up.

*   Don't turn on the television or make phone calls.

*   Don't evaluate your partner's performance or compare your lover to other partners you've had.

Instead:

*   Try some cuddling and snuggling.

*   Have a glass of wine together.

*   Take a bubble bath together.

*   Listen to music.

*   Brush each other's hair.

*   Scratch each other's backs.

*   Massage and caress each other.

*   Express your sexual feelings, thoughts, and desires.

*   Recharge and go at it again!

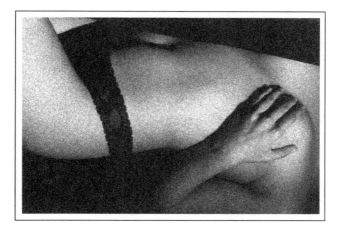

CHAPTER 12

Sacred Spots

What is the G-spot? What is the A-spot?

Where can you find them?

How do you stimulate them?

Do men have a G-spot?

Do women ejaculate?

Get geared up for a quick geography class. We're about to locate the most magical parts of your body—your erogenous zones. I'm talking about the spots on your body that are the hottest areas to hit—the ones that move mountains, trigger orgasmic eruptions, and set off geyser-sized ejaculations. These are the parts of the body that make you feel really out-of-control, "Yes! Yes! Yes!" head-banging-against-the-bedpost good. These are the spots on your body that feel so good that they can make sex, even safer sex, stellar. No joke. Sound good? Good. I'll start with the most well known of them all—the G-spot.

The G-Spot

Named after its original researcher, Ernest Gräfenberg, the **Gräfenberg spot**, better known as the "**G-spot**," is a small mass of erectile nerve tissue, ducts, glands, and blood vessels located between the pubic bone and the front of the cervix—about two inches in from the vaginal opening. Approximately the size of a pea, the G-spot varies in size and location, from dead center of the vaginal wall to an inch or so to the right or left of the center. When stimulated effectively, this area becomes engorged with blood and enlarges to about the size of a walnut. It is a sensitive area that does not lie directly on the vaginal wall, but can be felt through it. (**Note:** Not every woman is aroused by G-spot stimulation.)

WHY IS IT SUCH A HUGE DEAL?

If you've ever found this little piece of heaven or have been with a woman and found it, you know why the G-spot is such a big deal. It's like finding gold. A woman's world is rocked when this gold is mined, as Ashley knows:

"I am out of control when someone hits my G-spot! It usually happens when my partner and I are doing the missionary and are angled so that his penis is directly hitting my G-spot while one of us is stimulating my clitoris. That combination is absolutely incredible! I become such a screamer! You can't shut me up!"

Many women say that stimulation of this region allows them to not only experience one orgasm, but experience multiple orgasms on occasion as well. Ever since Dr. Beverly Whipple and Dr. John Perry announced their research findings on this most amazing erogenous zone back in the early 1980s, women and couples everywhere have been on a mission to find this bit of bliss.

FINDING THE G-SPOT

Shrouded in an aura of mystique, this elusive G-spot can be quite a task for a woman to find solo, unless she is in a sitting or squatting position. In either of these two positions, locating the G-spot can be more easily done with the help of a partner willing to play Indiana Jones.

Sarah enthusiastically tells us about how her partner found her G-spot:

I have one!! I wasn't sure at first, but I had read so much about it that I wanted to find out. So I asked my partner to poke around until he found it and—WOW! I am not an extremely vocal person in bed, but when he stimulates that spot, these uncontrollable screams and moans escape from my body.

He usually uses his fingers and stimulates it manually, although sometimes it takes a while and his arm gets very tired, but he says it's worth it because he loves listening to me! It's exactly how I read about it. At first, when the G-spot is stimulated, it feels like you have to pee, but if you can move past those few seconds, it is so worth it! It is the most intense orgasm(s) I have ever experienced!

The following are G-spot directions you ladies can pursue on your own or with a special someone. (If you go through all of these steps without any success, or if you think that the G-spot is the most over-rated thing since sliced bread, know that I presented this chapter pretty much so I could tell you about the G-spot and how to find it—not to make anybody feel bad.)

Don't get down or hung up on the fact that you can't find your (or your partner's) G-spot, or that you don't find stimulation of the spot very enjoyable. Everyone is different when it comes to their bodies and their erogenous zones. Some women don't respond to G-spot stimulation at all. Some women do, but don't find stimulating it all that grand. Still, other women find stimulation of the G-spot downright uncomfortable. So each to her own and enjoy whatever works for you!

How to Find Your G-Spot

1. Make sure your (and/or your partner's) nails are trimmed. If you must keep your long nails, you may want to put on latex gloves to cover up those claws! This is an area that you don't want to accidentally poke or scratch!

2. Urinate before you begin your exploration. That way, when you've found your G-spot, you may have the urge to pee but you can continue exploring, knowing your bladder is really empty. Within two to ten seconds of massaging the area, that initial "I gotta pee" feeling will be replaced by a strong, distinctive feeling of sexual pleasure.

3. Get aroused first. It's easier to find the G-spot if you're already sexually aroused, since the urethral sponge will swell and become more prominent. Plus, you'll enjoy your G-spot sensations more if you're already feeling stimulated. At some point while you're stimulating yourself, make sure you're in a squatting position or that you're sitting and leaning back. Both of these positions are the best to be in for effective solo exploration of the G-spot.

4. Insert a couple of your fingers, with your palm turned upward against the front wall of the vagina—about two inches in from the opening of the vagina on the front anterior wall (the one toward the stomach). Stroke the area, using firm pressure, and just explore that anterior wall. You should feel a slight swelling at the point where the G-spot is, anywhere from the size of a small bean to the size of a half-dollar.

5. If you have a partner helping you out, you may prefer to lie on your stomach with your hips slightly elevated and your legs apart. Once in this position, using two or three fingers, palm down, your partner should apply light, then firm pressure to the anterior wall by pressing down.

6. If you would prefer to be on your back (which actually makes finding the G-spot much more difficult), then you or your partner can insert a couple of fingers curved upwards, like a fish hook, before applying pressure in a "come hither" motion. Applying pressure and placing a second hand just above the pubic hairline on the

lower abdomen sometimes helps with G-spot stimulation while a female is on her back. For proper positioning, make sure that while on your back, your knees are bent and spread. Have your feet flat on the bed, with a small pillow under your buttocks.

7. Once you have located the G-spot area, slide your fingers from side to side, making the most of the middle finger. Apply a firm, upward pressure. Do this slowly, rhythmically pressing on the area. Move your pelvis to make contact with your fingers. All of this may result in twinges or contractions from your uterus. As you become more aroused, you (or your partner) once again have the option of placing the other hand over your pubic hair and slowly pressing.

8. Experiment with different amounts of pressure and finger movements. The G-spot is extremely sensitive to deep pressure and most women need firm pressure on the vaginal wall, with quick rhythm and a lot of friction, to have a G-spot orgasm. You can also try massaging motions and rocking your fingers, circling them around the front vaginal wall, always using a firm touch.

TIPS ON G-SPOT EXPLORATION

- ✳ Make sure that the vagina is well lubricated or else stimulation may not feel so stimulating!

- ✳ Using a diaphragm may interfere with G-spot stimulation in some women.

- ✳ Try using a dildo or G-spot vibrator if you're having difficulty locating and stimulating the spot.

- ✳ Mimic penile thrusting. Try thrusting your fingers in and out, in and out, exerting pressure upwards when withdrawing, to pleasure the G-spot.

- ✳ Lovers, once you've found the G-spot, try licking her clitoris at the same time. Or use your thumb to rub the clitoris while the fingers inside the vagina move in circles across the G-spot.

- ✳ For penis probing of the G-spot during intercourse, the woman-on-top and doggie-style are the best positions for stimulation. In the woman-on-top position, you may feel nothing or only slight pleasure the first time you try it. With practice in that position, you will experience greater G-spot stimulation.

Female Ejaculation

Female ejaculation is a phenomenon that has caused quite the fiasco on some couples' sheets and one that often occurs because of G-spot stimulation. Many women who experience female ejaculation during sex are quite embarrassed by it, usually because they think that they're urinating when it occurs. Their partners, usually thinking that their lovers have just peed on them, don't make the situation any easier, often making the women feel incompetent and unclean. Such reactions from both parties, to a very misunderstood female sexual response, can contribute to the female's suppression of orgasm. Such relationship stress and orgasm inhibition blows, since it's a situation that can be avoided entirely with a little bit of education.

> Female ejaculation is not a modern-day wonder. Even ancient cultures knew about it. The Indian Tantra, for example, considered ejaculate highly nutritious and called the fluid "amrita," meaning "divine nectar." It's actually only recently, however, that researchers have started investigating what female ejaculation actually is.

WHAT IS FEMALE EJACULATION?

Some women have prostatic tissue around their urethra—the Skene's glands—that expel a scentless fluid during orgasm. Often referred to as the "female prostate," these Skene's glands are similar to the male's prostate and produce this prostatic-like fluid, which is actually a blend of proteins similar to those in male seminal fluid. Bearing a resemblance to diluted skim milk, this fluid is *not* urine.

Many female ejaculators often experience the urge to ejaculate during sexual activity, especially when their G-spot is stimulated, but try to hold back for fear that they are going to urinate. Often, their partners think that this is the case as well. Those of you out there who thought that you were going to urinate or think that you have urinated should know that that isn't the case! You're just ejaculating—a perfectly normal, natural bodily function. It's nothing to be embarrassed about! After all, guys do it too.

Various studies have found that anywhere from 10 to 40 percent of females are ejaculators. Even those who are able to ejaculate do not ejaculate every time they have an orgasm. Amounts of fluid, for those who do ejaculate, also vary from just a few drops to a few tablespoons full.

A woman's partner may even feel the ejaculation during intercourse. It feels mostly as if he's getting sprayed with a water gun, with streams of fluid shooting on him in spurts. A male is likeliest to feel female ejaculation when the woman is on top, her warm fluid flowing down onto his penis. Reports from men who've experienced this say that it's quite erotic.

As long as people are aware of female ejaculation, it doesn't have to be embarrassing or shameful. It's actually a cool physiological response to sexual excitement. Yet, since so many people don't know about it, or understand what the ejaculated fluid really is, couples may want to talk about it before sexual relations take place so that there are no misunderstandings. Understanding female ejaculation helps women and couples to understand her sexual experience and responses and, if looked upon favorably, can even help to eroticize sex. For more information on female ejaculation, a good book is Deborah Sundahl's *Female Ejaculation and the G-Spot* (Hunter House, 2003).

So if you're a female ejaculator, talk to your partner about it. Chances are, he'll be intrigued and excited by this news. And it's a great way for you to show how turned on you get. If the amount of fluid being ejaculated is a real damper (no pun intended), those of you who may be heavy ejaculators but don't want to get the sheets all wet should lay down a towel before having sex.

The Male G-Spot

The prostate—that small gland just beneath the bladder—is the key to extremely intense male orgasms. It is the male G-spot and can be most effectively stimulated via the rectum.

Not so sure that you want to have somebody playing with your "exit-only" area? Some men claim that touching the prostate helps them to regain or maintain an erection, and some can orgasm solely from prostate stimulation. Prostate-induced orgasms are usually described as "full-bodied" and "deep."

STIMULATING THE PROSTATE

First, make sure that your nails are trimmed and that you're using *plenty* of lubrication. As with G-spot stimulation, some men like to have their prostate stimulated only once they're aroused. Anthony found this to be very true: "I've had my prostate stimulated. Early on, it has little effect for me, but it's really cool after I've been aroused for a while."

So go to town on yourself before you dive in. If you can, try to get your partner to get into it with you, too. Finding your prostate with a partner is always easier. To find your prostate

1. Lie on your back with your knees bent and your feet flat on the bed, or with your knees drawn up to your chest.

2. The most direct way for you or your partner to stimulate your prostate is by inserting a lubricated finger or thumb, preferably latex-gloved, about three inches into the anus.

3. Press against the front wall. The prostate will feel like a firm, rounded chestnut or a little dome.

4. Begin gently rubbing the prostate, fingers moving toward the front of the body. The initial pressure you will feel may trigger a sudden urge to urinate, followed by pleasurable sensations.

5. Gently stroke the gland in a downward direction and massage it, taking the time to occasionally move your fingers in and out of the anus. Make sure you keep pressing through the front wall of the rectum, about three inches in. When and if you do ejaculate, it will come in a gentle stream rather than in spurts.

Still not sure if you can or want to manually stimulate the prostate? Ladies, if your guy is willing, help him out here and show a little love. Some lovers may just need a little bit of encouragement from you to take your sex play to new, uncharted territory, like Geoffrey:

I've read about this male G-spot, and even how to find it on my own,
but I'm just not comfortable doing it. I have issues with anal stimulation,
but if I did it, I would probably have to be with a partner whom I
really trusted."

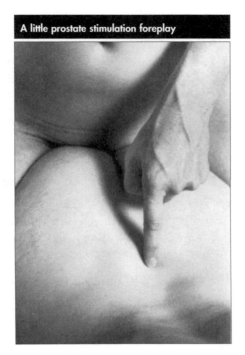

A little prostate stimulation foreplay

One way to make sure your partner is aroused is to play with and stroke his back and buttocks before stimulating him directly. For couples who would like to stimulate the prostate, but have issues with anal play, try pressing against his perineum with the ball of your thumb. For added effect, try massaging the penis as you stimulate the perineum or prostate. Furthermore, prostate stimulation is sometimes just the right touch for the perfect blow job.

The A-Spot

Ever wanted to get really wet during sex? To the point that you and your partner give "waterbed" a completely new meaning? Would you believe that one little erogenous zone can make your sex life wetter and better than it has ever been before?

If you don't know about it already, let me introduce you to the **anterior fornix erogenous (AFE) zone**, a.k.a. the "**A-spot.**" It is the smooth area midway between a woman's cervix and G-spot, on the anterior (front) wall of the vagina, that appears as a spongy, wrinkled, scrotal-like swelling and is extremely sensitive to stimulating touch. What makes this erogenous area so remarkable, so much more special than the other erogenous zones on a woman's body, is that the AFE zone has been found to play a role in vaginal lubrication.

In fact, this vaginal area is such a hidden treasure of vaginal lubrication that the A-spot's original researcher, Dr. Chua Chee Ann, has even developed the **AFE-zone stimulation technique**. This technique, targeting the A-spot, has been found to be beneficial to couples who experience vaginal dryness during sex and for couples who just want more natural vaginal lubrication during sexual activity. Best yet, the A-spot doesn't stop there! Research findings indicate that for some women the combination of vaginal lubrication and the A-spot's erotic sensitivity can result in orgasms.

THE AFE-ZONE STIMULATION TECHNIQUE

The AFE-zone stimulation technique is an arousal method that works as follows:

1. Ladies, you should be squatting or sitting and leaning back against a support, with your legs bent and pulled up toward your body.

2. You, or your partner, should insert an entire index finger into the vagina (use lube if you want to!).

3. With this index finger, gently stroke the inner half of the anterior vaginal wall.

4. Once lubrication begins, bring your finger out to stroke the spongy area that is at the outer half of the anterior vaginal wall, as well as the AFE zone. Use a long, repeated, in-and-out finger motion, moving up and down the entire length of the anterior vaginal wall, for the best results.

Note that for her body to become increasingly stimulated by this method, the technique should be practiced daily for at least one week, about 5–10 minutes each time. Over time, she'll hopefully experience greater lubrication and perhaps even orgasm.

Your Erogenous Zones

While stimulation of the G-spot, A-spot, or prostate can provide hours of quality entertainment, don't ignore the rest of your body! Your body is covered with erogenous zones. You're practically one big erogenous zone! So consider other parts of your body that might be particularly sensitive to sexual stimulation. Once you've found them, stroke them. Stimulate them. Have your partner indulge in them.

Among the more popular erogenous zones, besides the genitals, are your lips, breasts, neck, thighs, back, ears, stomach, feet, ear lobes, and scalp. So try nibbling hungrily on his neck. Try darting your tongue in and out of her ear. Try playfully nipping his ear lobe. Try firmly massaging her toes, concentrating on the skin between the toes, soles, and arches. Stroke and kiss his chest and nipples. Gently bite at her lips, then run your tongue lasciviously over them. Suck on his fingers. There are tons of erogenous zones to choose from. You may find them in the most unexpected places.

No matter what the erogenous zone, all of them are fair game for safer sex, if the two of you even feel that you still have the energy for sex after erogenous zone stimulation! You and your partner may be so satiated from "smurfing" your erogenous zones that other forms of sex, like vaginal intercourse, don't need to be pursued. G-spot, A-spot, and prostate gland stimulation are definitely the way to keep things wet, wild, and wonderful without necessarily "going all the way." They're as gratifying as intercourse because they produce many of the same results as sexual intercourse—a nice thing to keep in mind when you're trying to figure out just how physical you want to get with your partner.

If you're looking for ways to make sex with a condom hot, erogenous zones are definitely areas of the body worth exploring. They're body parts that, when stimulated, can help eroticize safer sex and that can improve your technique and make you a better lover. Daydream with me for a minute here...

The condom is on and you're making steamy, luscious love. You're alternating between shallow and deep thrusts, all the while targeting that exquisite G-spot. Aww yeah, you hear some moaning—loud moaning—now. The juices are flowing, and your bodies are trembling, and you're furiously pumping, and then a finger gives the prostate some rhythmic pressure. There's gasping, bodies arching, legs and arms intertwined and squeezing, and "Ohhh, baby!" and the two of you climax—HARD! Don't forget that you have a condom to take off after withdrawal.

CHAPTER 13

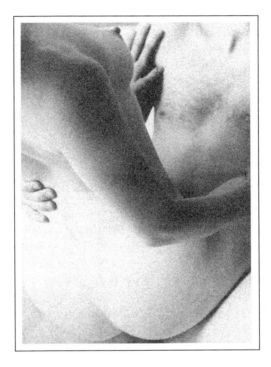

Talk Dirty to Me

What can you say when you want to talk dirty?

What is the role of sound in sex?

What are some hot things you can say during phone sex?

Dirty talk is one of those tantalizing, provocative, slightly soulful sexual instruments that puts stains on your sheets and beat to your banging. Either you want it or you don't. It can either totally spoil the mood or make it absolutely mind-blowing. I prefer to think that it caters more toward the latter, and it *really* eroticizes safer sex.

Talking dirty is one of those sexual enhancers that can make a partner want you *more* because you're telling your lover how much you want him, how much you adore her, how much that person turns you on. Plus, it's a great sensual aid in that people love hearing nice things about themselves. Talking dirty appeals to the narcissist in all of us. People love being told when something they're doing feels good, how sexy they are, and how you can't get enough of them. After all, who can resist flattery?

Oops, Am I Bad?

Talking dirty always seems like one of those taboo things you only read about in *Penthouse Forum,* or you hear people saying to each other in porns. That's part of what makes it seem so racy, so bad, so…so…erotic. Talking dirty can be a hard thing to do because it is just that—talking dirty. If you're normally a polite, respectable person, which most of us like to think we are, it can be hard to imagine yourself being capable of saying "nasty" things, especially to a lover. I mean, what if he thinks you're being slutty? Or what if she thinks you're being disrespectful? Or what if your lover finds it more of a turn-off than a turn-on?

Part of being able to talk dirty is being willing to take a chance on it, being willing to take the risk of what it can do for you and your partner, and seeing where it can take you. If it's easier, think of it as "erotic talk" or "sexy talk" because that doesn't sound as bad. Part of doing it is getting into that frame of mind. At any rate, talking dirty can add just the right touch to almost any safer sexual encounter, as discovered by Ashton:

I remember the first time I tried talking dirty. I pushed all inhibitions aside and just tried it. My partner was most attentive, hanging on every word. I noticed that his breathing changed to these deep, hard shudders and his muscles tensed as I became more heated and more animated in telling him what I wanted and how much he was turning me on. Naturally, I threw in the occasional "bad" word to make it dirty, and you know what? He was digging it; he almost didn't believe that it was my first time doing it.

So the moral of that story is: Trust your ability to be able to talk dirty. Give it a chance! Even the purest of the pure have it in them to "be bad," including you!

Learning How to Talk Dirty

PART I: WHAT TO SAY

A lot of people talk dirty during sex—65 percent of men and 63 percent of women to be exact. Sometimes, remembering those figures is just the right kind of encouragement you'll need to tap into your natural, talking dirty talents.

One way you can become more comfortable talking dirty to your lover is if you can talk erotically to yourself, especially while you masturbate. You may have to work at this, starting with simply making sounds.

Eventually, you can start to quietly say a few things to yourself or to whomever you're fantasizing about talking to at the moment, e.g., whispering, "Make me come!" If you want to get completely carried away with your practice session, try moaning and groaning between utterances. Eventually, you'll be able to work this stuff into your lovemaking.

Now, I don't know if the following are statements that you would necessarily want to say to a partner. I'm simply laying them out to give you a few ideas. In talking dirty, you have to find what you're comfortable saying and to whom. Different people are receptive to different terms. Some are a little more hard-core than others. What you may have been able to say to a former partner, you may not be able to say to a new one. So keeping all of those factors in mind, here are some things you might want to say in talking dirty...

✳   "You make me soooo hard."

✳   "I want to make your pussy throb."

✳   "Do you want to tie me down?" (Say this one only if you mean it.)

✳   "You make me soooo horny!"

✳   "I love your body!"

✳   "Let your juicy, probing tongue work my cock."

✳   "I want you. No—I *need* you!"

✳   "I want to feel you inside of me." "I want to *feel* you." (Those are *killer*.)

✳   "You make me *so* hot."

✳   "Do I make you think nasty thoughts?"

✳   "Put your face between my thighs."

✳   "Spank me."

✳   "I want your fresh, aching beast slamming in me."

✳   "Go 'head, Daddy."

Now those are just a few suggestions to get you started. I'm hoping that you can go nuts coming up with some stuff on your own. In case you're not feeling that creative or don't know if you have that erotica writer vocabulary in you, here are some hot words to keep in mind to help you out. Try regularly incorporating any of the following racy verbs and you'll be talking like a porn star in heat in no time:

COMBINE RACY VERBS...

lick	tease	screw	squeeze	suck	play
eat	rub	fondle	caress	grab	kiss
blow	nibble	touch	bite	chew	push
pull	stick	ram	smell	hump	thrust
swallow	drink				

Combine these verbs with some of the following colorful adjectives and you're golden:

... WITH COLORFUL ADJECTIVES				
aching	erect	raging	hungry	tight
big	wet	stiff	swollen	juicy
soft	hot	sweet	nasty	hard
firm	luscious	steamy	naked	massive

Phew! I'm fanning myself. What wonderful, delicious words—they're *so* loaded! Anyway, that should almost be enough for you, but we won't stop there. We want your lover screaming, *"More!!!"* Of course all of this talk becomes even dirtier with all of those lovely, slang names we have for genitalia in the English language. Most people are not crazy about most of these words, probably because they're so "dirty." However, in the right context, during the right moment, with the right person, these words can be just what you need to talk dirty. (And you know, don't you, that these are, by far, not all of them!)

VAGINA	PENIS	BREASTS
muff	dick	boobs
cunt	cock	hooters
pussy	woody	tits
beaver	willy	jugs
booty	family jewels	melons
hole	prick	rack
snatch	dong	knockers
bush	johnson	chest
cooter	gun	bosom
twat	member	buds
flower	beast	
blossom		

Hopefully that's enough to get you started or recharged talking dirty. If you need some more help with this kind of talk, go to your local bookstore or convenience store and buy a dirty magazine or novel—guaranteed to give you a few ideas.

PART II: GOING FOR IT

As I said before, people like different means of communicating with one another, and they also dig different words as far as getting all sexed-up and talking dirty. We all have our own comfort zones when it comes to what kinds of sexy stuff we like to hear—and *when*, for that matter. Like Karl, a 25-year-old public relations coordinator, told me:

> I like moaning, but not when it's too much or too exaggerated. Don't be an actress. One time I had a girl and it was like out of a porno with "Fuck me hard!" and I just started to laugh.... I like the girl to be quiet if people are around. She needs to be aware of her surroundings and discreet about what she's doing. If nobody can hear us, then it's a different story. But there needs to be some self-restraint if others can hear.

When working dirty talk into your sex life, start easy and feel out the language your partner is receptive to. You may even find that the two of you prefer not to use four-letter words or genitalia slang in getting your juices flowing, and that's fine. So to avoid getting slapped, emotionally bruising your partner, or getting laughed at by a lover like Karl, you probably want to ask beforehand what sexual terms your partner finds arousing or unappealing.

Once the modes of acceptable, "proper" communication have been established, you may want to begin, for instance, by telling her, "I suck my tongue when I think of going down on your swollen, aching twat." If she can handle that, work up to something a little racier, "I want your sopping-wet cunt humping my face while I tongue-fuck you." This may be a bit of a leap for some of you, I know, but I trust that you can work your way up to it just fine with LOTS of practice.

Even a *little* bit of dirty talk can do wonders for your sex life. It's a great way of grabbing your protection and turning it into a very sexy activity. Just imagine all of the things you could whisper in his ear as you slide the condom down over his penis. Think of all of the enticing things you can murmur to her, telling her what you're going to do to her, as you roll the condom down over your shaft. Pretty hot scenario.

Dirty Talk and Fantasy

If all of this talking dirty so far isn't hard-core enough for you or if you're looking for a sheet-rippin' good time, you can work to a point where, if you know your partner's favorite erotic fantasies, you can incorporate them into talking dirty during sex. For example, if you know he's into having a sexual encounter that involves more than just the two of you, you could say, "I want to blow you while someone else fucks me from behind" or "Do you want to watch me do someone else?"

Granted, you may not ever want to do either of these things, but they're very sexy. Plus, he'll have about a bazillion erotic thoughts racing through his head as the two of you are messing around that are going to make the jizz fly and his motor roar like you've never known it to before.

If your partner doesn't seem crazy about incorporating such fantasy talk into your sex life at first, point out that this kind of talking dirty would be a great way to eroticize safer sex, that it could help make putting on the protection and going at it really hot. Hopefully, your partner will see—or should I say hear—talking dirty as a crafty tool to be used at least on occasion, and after reading this chapter, you'll be showing your lover how it's done. Talking dirty is a way of toying with thoughts that your relationship would never pursue, plus it acts as a way of eroticizing sex while keeping it safe.

Just Make Some Noise!

THE ROLE OF SOUND IN SEX

Sometimes less is more and that can be true when it comes to choosing between talking dirty or making simpler sounds. Erotic moans and murmurs can be *such* a turn-on. Even the slightest bit of noise from your partner, aside from the various ways your body enjoys naturally expelling gas, during sexual activity enhances it. So if you're excited, stimulated, ready to explode…let your partner know. Groan if something she does feels good. Let your breathing get heavy and take your "ooo's" and "ah'uh, ah'uh" up an octave, like a squeaky toy doll, when he's rocking your world.

If you really can't contain yourself and need to make even more noise than that, get loud and theatrical—let loose and exaggerate your state of frenzied ecstasy. Show your gratitude. Unleash your undying passion. Shrieks, squeals, and moans not only excite your lovers, but reassure them that they're pleasuring you too. Tristan, a 20-year-old student, prefers partners who make noise:

> I find it a real turn-on when a woman moans or talks during sex. When she does this, she makes me feel like I am doing something right and that she is enjoying the experience. If someone is silent, on the other hand, it is a real turn-off to me. It makes me feel inadequate and really makes me consider whether or not I would like to continue.

People like sound during intercourse. When they're getting it on, they don't want to feel like they're in a silent film—they like noise! Madison is into it:

> One of my favorite hook-ups ever was a heated make-out session during which my partner made little moans between kisses, and especially when I worked my tongue into his ear. Granted, such making out led to other, slightly more intimate activities, but that prelude is among the top in my book and sticks out because he is one of the few guys I've known who has had the balls to make some noise!

DON'T SOUND LIKE A BROKEN RECORD

Sound check—a warning to make sure that talking dirty doesn't put a damper on your sex life: Make sure that you don't always sound the same or say the same thing every time you have sex. I had a roommate once who was rather vocal during sex, so the rest of us in the apartment always knew when she was getting some. While embarrassing and somewhat interesting to overhear at first, as the school year progressed, her "Oh's!" and "Yes!" and "Ah's!" and "Oh God!" soon became really old and even boring. It was always the same thing, *every* single time. It got to the point that I started to feel sorry for her boyfriend who, by the way, was feeling that their love life was rather stagnant. Gee, I wonder why.

THERE'S SOMETHING TO BE SAID FOR QUIET

Oh, and another thing, it's okay to be quiet on occasion, too. Sometimes it adds to the sense of peace and comfort you have in simply becoming intimate with your partner. Quiet allows you to enjoy all of the other sounds that you might not always get to appreciate, that of skin on skin, slow breathing that becomes gasping, and sheets crinkling. In addition, quiet sexual encounters can be especially appealing for those times that you or your partner may want to fantasize about being with somebody else. Hearing too much can make such a mental escape a bit difficult.

Phone Sex

Phone sex is a nice alternative to talking dirty or a means through which you can talk dirty. Phone sex is safe sex that can be romantic, nasty, or anything in-between. It can be a splendiferous substitute for lovers in a long-distance relationship or a way to add a kick to your daily routine. (Note that I'm not talking about obscene phone calls—illegal calls in which the person you're talking to hasn't given consent to such a phone conversation.)

Topanga, who's in a long-distance relationship, is among those who have come to appreciate phone sex over talking dirty:

> I don't know how I feel about talking dirty. I had been in a relationship where the guy and I did it all the time. It got to the point that that's all he ever wanted to do during sex and it got to be demeaning and demanding. He wouldn't have sex unless I talked dirty to him. So I'm not doing that anymore. I do like phone sex, however. It doesn't have to get dirty. Plus, phone sex is the best when you masturbate!

Topanga brings up a good point, taking phone sex to a whole, new level—that of masturbating. So if you haven't already, take Topanga's lead. Try masturbating yourself while on the phone with your partner, with or without the dirty talk. Touch yourself as you normally would and, in great detail, tell your lover what you're doing, "I'm playing with my head right now and it's all wet with pre-cum..." or "I'm slowly reaching between my legs, gliding my fingers through my juices.... Ahhhh—now I'm massaging my nipples with...oh...it's so slippery!"

You might even have fun telling your partner what to do, "Rub your cock faster! Harder!" or "Take off your bra.... Now your panties.... Slide your fingers over your clit.... Rub...."

The two of you can also pretend that you *really are* with each other having sex, "You're in me! (pant) Harder...Yeah (pant, pant)...Oh God! (pant, pant, pant)...I'm coming!...(orgasmic scream)" or "I'm thrusting my meat between your perky mounds. Squeeze them around my shaft while I titty-fuck you!"

You can also pretend that you're total strangers getting off on each other. Other alternatives to phone sex are talking about what you're going to do to each other the next time you get together, or pretending that one of you is a sex-worker.

If talking dirty isn't your partner's thing, you can do things to make up for the lack of such magic in your sex life. Try putting on music that is a bit raw. Or incorporate a porn video as part of foreplay and keep it running while you're messing around. Get carried away in Peter North or Jenna Jameson's Academy Award–worthy screams and cries of passion!

CHAPTER 14

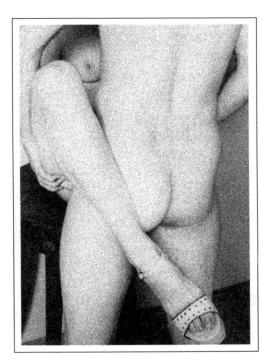

You Want Something to Play With?

What are some must-have sex toys?

How do I incorporate sex toys into my sex life?

Sex Toys

"I'm all about sex toys. Cock rings with vibrators, anal vibrators, ben wa balls, massage toys, oils, things that get hot when you blow on them, scented oils.... I have an entire chest full of sex toys. I'm always looking for something new, a new experience. They're great!"

Haywood Jay is one of many who has indulged himself with sex toys. His quote reflects the attitude most people our age have toward sex—one of adventure—and sex toys definitely bring out the adventurer in all of us. While people may normally think of sex toys as being those kinky "play things" we see in sex shops, a **sex toy** can be any object that's used to enhance sexual pleasure.

Perhaps some of you have thought about how sex toys could spice up things between the sheets and enhance your safer-sex experience. Sex toys are great because they add variety to sexual activity that doesn't need to involve intercourse, and they make any sex act so exciting that you and your partner are not going to be bothered by the fact that you're using protection. As long as you use them properly, sex toys are handy, erotic tools for safer sex.

My friend Beth and I had the best time collecting the juice for this chapter! We hit a sex shop and just took our time strolling around—for research purposes, of course. We even talked to the guy behind the counter to find out about best-selling items.

The following are some of the sex toys we came across, plus some other ideas for eroticizing safer sex.

Anal Beads

Ideal for the nerve endings in the anus and for prostate massage, **anal beads** are usually five plastic or latex beads, strung together on a nylon or cotton cord that has a ring at the end. The beads can range in size from as small as marbles to as big as golf balls, with 1 to 1½-inch balls being the most popular.

Anal beads

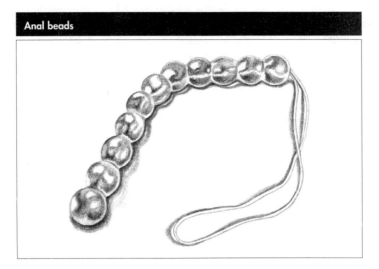

To use anal beads, first use lots of lube on your partner's rectum and on the beads. Then insert one bead at a time. Not only does this give the anus time to adjust to each bead, but it intensifies the feeling of the rectum around each bead as well.

Tip: Anal bead play can be made even better if you stimulate your lover's genitals as you're inserting the beads.

Remember that insertion is only half the fun. Anal beads can be as much of a pleasure to pull out as they are to put in. You can pull them out as your partner is climaxing or wait until after your partner has had an orgasm. Make sure you withdraw the beads *slowly* and *gently*.

One concern people have about anal beads is how to keep them clean. Some people put a condom over the beads and knot the open end of the condom. That way, all they have to do is throw away the condom and rinse off the beads. Users have also found that nylon strings and latex beads are the best to use as far as cleanliness goes, since the soft or jelly rubber beads are hard to disinfect.

Warning: Never substitute random objects, like ping-pong balls or golf balls, when engaging in anal play. I doubt that any of you want to deal with the embarrassment of landing in the emergency room with a foreign object lodged up your ass.

Note: Ben wa balls are solid metal balls that can be used for anal stimulation or placed in the vagina and used in the same way as anal beads.

With any sex toy, it's a good idea to use a water-based lubricant, but this is an especially good idea with an anal sex toy since the rectum does not produce any natural lubricant of its own.

Blindfolds

Tie a blindfold (you can use a scarf or tie) around your partner's eyes. This element of trust can make sexual arousal quite intriguing and can heighten anticipation. By not relying on sight to process the sexual experience, your partner is forced to tap into other senses and sensations that are normally ignored. Her skin comes alive. His heartbeat picks up a pace. The sound of the crackling condom wrapper means something big is about to happen! Anything could happen! The air is dripping with anticipation!

Geoffrey loved a blindfold session that he once had: "I teased my ex-girlfriend once with a strawberry while she was blindfolded. I ran it under her nose and played with it on her lips, but I wouldn't let her have it. I had heated Nutella, so I could dip the strawberry in it. It was really great. She loved it...."

Body Paints

Take art to another form. Get some water-based paints and turn your bodies into each other's canvases and then each other's masterpieces. Enjoy how slick and smooth the paint feels as you create designs and messages like "I love you" on your lover. Even finger painting in kindergarten was never quite as good as this!

Butt Plugs

Whether a butt plug has stimulating ripples or is baby smooth, this toy can be divine to insert or pull out. Whether vinyl, silicone, or rubber, butt plugs come in a variety of sizes and are usually diamond-shaped, with a narrow tip and flared base (which helps to make sure it doesn't go in any farther than it's supposed to). Silicone is the most resilient option, retains body heat, and is easy to clean. The main pleasure people get out of butt plugs is enjoying the sensation of just having it there. So try having one of you slip a plug into place while the other one puts on a condom. Or have one

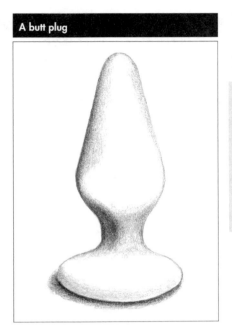

A butt plug

handy to heighten the sensations of protected sex by slipping it in while your partner is climaxing.

How to Clean Your Sex Toys

Use warm water, a mild soap, and a moistened cloth to clean the toy. Allow it to completely dry before storing it in a cool and dry place. Proper care of your sex toys can help prevent undesirable bacterial growth.

Cameras

Can you think of a project that could be any more fun than making your very own, personal porn video? Not sure if it's something that you're into? Take some encouragement from Maya, who is all for making your own sex movies:

> The fantasy about videotaping sex stems from the fact that, deep down, we all believe we're as erotic and photogenic as the greatest porn star. The great thing about actually taping ourselves is discovering, Hey, we really are!!

> Sex itself is so erotic that even the most bumbling couple can generate lust when seen writhing naked across a TV screen. Plus, who doesn't want to be their partner's favorite porn star? Women love videotaping sex because no flat hair or flabby thighs can keep them from looking utterly erotic and sensual. Men love it because, well, it's related to sex.

Tip: Make sure that when you're doing this, you use a wide shot, which allows you to see a lot more action. You also don't want the video camera up too close, since this could make the overall focus more difficult as well.

The nice thing about home video porn is that you get to be the actor or actress, so it's the perfect excuse for you to try things you might not normally do. Dress up in skimpy, slutty lingerie. Dig out that leopard

G-string you use only on special occasions. Go heavier on the make-up. Sport a condom, just like the modern-day porno stars. Lather yourselves up in body oil. Put on a costume. Throw on those f.m. (fuck me) heels you hardly ever wear. The two of you will be erecting a porn star in no time!!

Not digging the directing of a home video? Then strike a pose. When people ask me what would make for a great Valentine's Day present, I always tell them a Polaroid camera. What's sexier, more personal, and gives you and your partner more potential than that? It's hours of entertainment that the two of you can enjoy. Ewan is one of the many who has played photographer:

> I've taken nude pictures with my girlfriend. The first time I did it was when we were in Atlantic City for a weekend. We were sitting in the motel room with nothing to do. We were playing strip poker and I was winning every hand. She was buck naked and I had a camera, so I was like, "Let's take some pictures."

Note (and this is an important one): While the videotaping or taking pictures of you and your partner can certainly make for future swoon-inducing, energy-sapping sex sessions, be careful with this erotica. If you and your partner decide to take snapshots of each other, make sure you keep the negatives of yourself. If you go the route of videotaping yourselves, it's a really good idea to erase this video soon afterward in case your relationship goes awry. If you don't, weeks, months, years later it could make you sweat when you surf the Web or when you run for president.

Cock Rings

Hey, men, want to stay harder longer? Want to heighten your sense of arousal? Longing for a sense of firmness and control when erect? A cock ring may be just what you're looking for.

A **genital ring** (**cock ring**) is a metal or latex object that fits over the base of the penis or around the entire penis and scrotum. Leather straps with snaps or Velcro models are available as well. Such an object turns you into quite the charger because it sensitizes your penis to natural erogenous surfaces by, supposedly, partially "trapping" the blood that has made the penis erect.

Warning: Be sure to purchase the real thing and use it carefully. *Never* try to use stuff that might be readily available to you, like rubber bands,

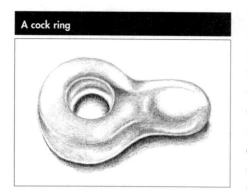

A cock ring

strings, or wires, to achieve the same sense of pressure on the penis. Such homemade imitations of genital rings may cause physical damage and pain, and may dangerously impede the normal flow of blood to the penis and could cause an aneurysm. Always use commercially available products that are specifically made for this kind of sexual enhancement. Also, make sure that you are using a proper-sized cock ring, one that is loose enough to allow semen to ejaculate. One that is too small could cause irreparable damage by forcing the semen back into the prostate.

Comb/Brush

Brush each other's hair. It feels so good to have your hair brushed and to have the bristles sensually massage your scalp. If you're in the mood, you can move south and brush each other's pubic hair. With just a razor and a pair of scissors, you can move on to pubic art. Have a good time trimming each other's pubic hair, shaving a design, or going bald down there completely.

Dildos

A **dildo** is an object, often designed to look like an artificial, erect penis, made of rubber, silicone, or latex that can be inserted into the vagina or anus and that, unlike the vibrator, doesn't vibrate. It is a toy that has been used by both sexes for thousands of years. Silicone is the most expensive type to buy, but it is also the easiest to clean, is more resilient, and retains heat, plus it becomes more flexible with time and use.

Dildos come in a wide range of sizes, colors, textures, and styles. Some dildos are straight, others are curved in order to stimulate the G-spot.

Thus, in shopping for one, you need to consider the length, thickness, hardness, and texture you would not only enjoy, but could handle as well.

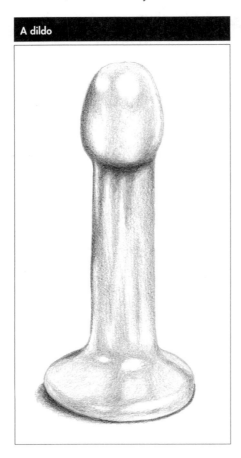

A dildo

Dildos can be used during masturbation or with a partner. The main pleasure derived from a dildo is the mere feeling of it or moving it in a thrusting motion.

Dildos can also be worn strapped on with a harness (they are about a half-inch shorter once in the harness). The possibilities of sex play with harnessed dildos are many. For example, among heterosexuals a dildo harness may be used by the female to anally thrust her male partner, or by the male to stimulate the female's vagina and anus at the same time.

Traditional harnesses come in two basic styles, with either a center strap running between the legs or with a leg strap encircling the thigh. They are available in leather or in a washable fabric. For women who want clitoral stimulation while wearing a harness, a vibrating cock ring or pearl can be slipped between the body and the harness.

> Never swap sex toys with somebody unless they have been properly cleaned first. Also, make sure you never use a toy anally and then vaginally without proper cleaning since this can introduce the vagina to bacteria and viruses that may cause some unpleasant health problems.

Feathers and Fur

Ooooh là là! Add some tactile sensation to your sex life and stimulate the body's biggest organ—your skin! Use items, like feathers or fur, to tickle your lover's fancy, slowly going over her erogenous zones or rubbing certain muscle-shuddering parts of his body.

Handcuffs

Made of fur, metal, or leather, handcuffs or restraints can be where it's at. Clip your lover's wrists or ankles together, put a condom on your "prisoner" if needed, and go nuts. Mercy!

Liberator Shapes

This fun new line of "bedroom adventure gear" is all about angles and trying new positions. Sold in wedge, ramp, stage, or cube form, these supportive, cushy shapes allow for greater intimacy, deeper penetration, better thrust power, and improved G-spot stimulation. Whether for anal, oral, or vaginal-penile sex, you're in for a wild new sexual experience, with the shapes providing comfort and doing half the work for you!

Old T-Shirts

Give an old T-shirt a little bit of life one last time. Put it on your partner, then rip it off—with your teeth!

Vibrators

Many couples have introduced a third party to their sex life—a vibrator! The **vibrator** is a handheld device that vibrates and stimulates your nerves to produce a pleasant sensation. It is a toy primarily used to enhance sexual responsiveness and sexual pleasure, with or without a partner. Some are shaped like a penis, while others are shaped like a high-powered club—wand-style—for massaging not only the genitals, but the whole body as well. Coil-type vibrators are also available, with soft latex or plastic heads and attachments. You can buy vibrators in many styles; an assortment of colors (even glow-in-the-dark); either battery operated, rechargeable, or with a cord. Some vibrators have adjustable speeds and attachments.

Vibrators should be properly looked after and kept away from water (unless they're waterproof) when switched on.

HOW TO USE A VIBRATOR

Vibrators can be used on women to stimulate the clitoris, mons area, and anus, or they can be inserted into the vagina. The most common movement in using a vibrator is a back and forth or up and down movement, with a circular-type movement being commonly used as well. Some women think it feels terrific to move the vibrator around their clitoris while rock-

ing their pelvis in an easy-going "thrusting" motion. For those who know how to use their PC muscle (see next chapter), it can be fun to rhythmically squeeze this muscle while rocking forward and relaxing it while rocking back.

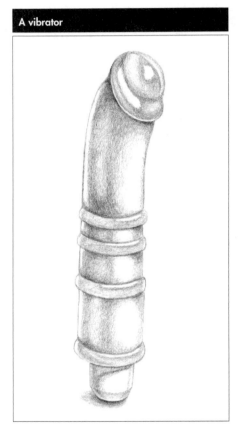

A vibrator

Women who are a little more advanced in vibrator use, and who want to make things even more mind-blowing, can do all of this while breathing rhythmically. An expert vibrator user may even place a nice dildo into the vagina and then move it with one hand in rhythm to her pelvic and PC movements. This further enhances the feel of the vibrator that her other hand is using on her clitoris.

Most women who use vibrators report that orgasms triggered by vibrator stimulation are more intense, and nearly half of them experience multiple orgasms when using a vibrator. The secret to multiple clitoral orgasms with a vibrator is to back off on the pressure from time to time. If pressure is applied for too long, the clitoris can become a bit desensitized, almost numb, but only temporarily. In that case, keep the vibrator moving and avoid direct contact with the clitoris until the energy builds back up again.

About 72 percent of couples use a vibrator while engaging in sexual activity with their partner. Either the woman stimulates herself with it while her partner holds and strokes her, or the partner just watches her get off with it, or he stimulates her with it himself. Sometimes partners try to hold the vibrator in a position where both of them can be stimulated genitally at the same time. The vibrating sensation can also be quite pleasurable for men.

> Vibrators can be also be used to stimulate a male's genitals, particularly the tip of his penis or the area between the testicles and anus (the perineum), or his anus.

So go ahead—try some of these toys! Turn your bedroom into a little safer-sex playground!!

RESOURCES

To check out or order sex toys, call or visit the following:

Adam and Eve catalog: (800) 274-0333 or www.adameve.com

Toys in Babeland: www.babeland.com

Eve's Garden: (800) 848-3837 or www.evesgarden.com

Good Vibrations: (800) 289-8423 or www.goodvibes.com

Liberator Shapes: www.liberatorshapes.com

CHAPTER 15

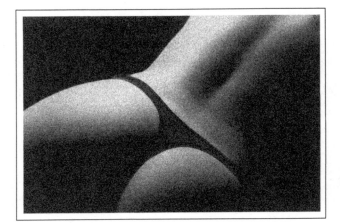

Y-Bo
with Y-vonne

What is the PC muscle?

What are the benefits of PC-muscle control?

How do I do Kegel exercises?

Why would I want to do Kegels?

Are there Kegel exercises for men that help with ejaculatory control?

She tightened her muscle around his shaft, her vaginal walls clutch-
ing and massaging it as his breathing became faster, more shallow.
She felt another surge of her vaginal juices flow through her canal
and she clenched her muscles around his penis, again and again,
harder and harder. As she consciously applied pressure and
squeezed, he groaned and twisted in convulsions of pleasure, wanting
it to never end.

Wish you could do this to your lover during sex? Wish she could do it to you? It isn't a daydream or erotic fiction. It could happen. You could make it happen. I'm going to tell you how. The key to it all is a little bit of Y-BO work, discipline, dedication, and the training of those south-of-the-border pelvic-floor muscles—namely your PC muscle. My what???

The PC Muscle

The **pubococcygeus muscle (PC muscle)** is a group of pelvic-floor muscles that are attached to the pelvic bone and act as your reproductive system's hammock, holding in your pelvic organs. It runs from the pubic bone to the tailbone, encircling the base of your penis or vagina, urethra, and rectum. It naturally contracts when you orgasm.

Your **pudendal nerve**, which runs through this muscle, triggers most of the PC muscle's reactions. This nerve detects most genital and anal stimulation and sends such signals to your brain. This nerve also transmits signals from the brain to the PC muscle, inducing the rhythmic contractions that are associated with the most common types of orgasm.

In the 1940s, Dr. Arnold Kegel developed **Kegel** (pronounced *KAY-gul*) **exercises**, which work the floor of the pelvic muscles, to help women who suffer from *urinary incontinence* (a condition in which urine leaks from the urethra during coughing, laughing, and/or sexual arousal). It was soon discovered that these exercises also ultimately increase pleasure during intercourse, increase sexual desire, intensify orgasms, and can help one become multi-orgasmic. They do so because they exercise the muscles that you use during orgasm. Like any of your body's muscles, the PC muscle becomes more responsive as it's toned. The more toned it is, the greater the increase in your sexual arousal and sensation.

BENEFITS OF KEGEL EXERCISES FOR WOMEN

I'm sensing that your mind keeps wandering, that you can't stop thinking about all of the potential these exercises might hold for your sex life. With vaginal muscle strength equivalent to the suction power of a Swedish penis enlarger, you're seeing making love in a whole new light. Suddenly, with this new, killer grip during sex, your guy becomes your prey. And you're *loving* it, fellows, practically crying, "Don't be careful, baby—squeeze!" every time you get laid. It's magnificent!

At any rate, I must warn you that exposing you to this information is probably going to raise the stakes in your relationships as far as good sex goes. It might even change the whole dating and pick-up scene, and your attitude toward partner qualifications at that, forever. Perhaps one day, instead of hearing, "What's your sign?" at a bar or party, you'll get, "So how strong is your PC muscle?" or "Feel like showing me some of your Kegels later?"

The PC muscle is the muscle everybody loves because everyone benefits from it. Yet while Kegel exercises are beneficial for both men and women, the benefits are a little more plentiful for the females. For you ladies, Kegel exercises will

✳   make it easier for you to reach not only orgasm, but multiple
     orgasms too

* make your orgasms stronger and better

* make your vagina more sensitive so you feel more when penetrated. His penis feels much better and bigger inside you when you squeeze

* give you a tighter-feeling vagina

* give you more sexual self-confidence during sexual activity

* support the bladder, helping to preventing the leaking of urine when you sneeze or cough (especially after childbirth)

* aid in proper placement of the diaphragm

* help reduce the chance of vaginal infections, by bringing an increased blood supply to the vaginal lining

* make childbirth much easier

Because PC-muscle exercises promise such amazing results, you'll find yourself increasingly interested in sex. Plus, not only will you score from doing Kegel exercises, your lover will too. If you do Kegels, he will notice a tremendous difference in your tightness—you'll be able to pull and squeeze his penis better—and he'll also enjoy your stronger, sturdier vagina. Ultimately, due to these exercises, both you and your partner will enjoy greater participation in sex and more sexual satisfaction.

BENEFITS OF KEGEL EXERCISES FOR MEN

Men should know that Kegel exercises are not just a girl thing. Since two to three inches of your penis are rooted in the PC muscle, your sex muscle, you can gain a lot from these exercises as well. If you can increase your PC-muscle strength, you can learn to separate your orgasms from ejaculation and become multi-orgasmic. Since male orgasm builds from the prostate, the PC-muscle strength around this gland is essential in your ability to control orgasms. Furthermore, such muscle control prevents hardening and swelling of the prostate. If you practice your own PC-muscle exercises, they can benefit you, too, and you will see the following results:

✳ They can help you become multi-orgasmic!

✳ With increased pelvic-floor muscle awareness, they help delay and control orgasm.

✳ You will have better, longer lasting erections.

✳ You will have a shorter refractory period.

✳ The intensity of your orgasm will increase—with a more pleasurable, forceful ejaculation.

✳ Your energy following an orgasm will increase and you won't be as tired.

✳ Your prostate will stay healthy and your risk of prostate cancer may be reduced.

Word is that, ultimately, after practicing Kegel exercises, you'll have such incredible PC-muscle strength that you'll be able to perform the "towel trick." If your PC muscle is healthy, you will amaze everyone by hanging a small towel over your erect penis and willfully raising it up and down by contracting that muscle. Forget the DJ! How's that for party entertainment?

Identify Your PC Muscle

This is all pretty good stuff, I'd say, and you're probably sold on these exercises, too. You want to train every day, sticking with this workout plan as you have no other. You're going to have the best sex ever, going to be the best lover ever, going to have to…find out where those muscles are, exactly.

Not to take anything away from Dr. Kegel, but this is where this chapter becomes Y-BO because I get to be trainer. Anyway, I think you'll like my Y-BO workout, too, because there's no sweat, none of that no-pain-no-gain exercise, and no diet component whatsoever. Sounds almost too good to be true, but it's not! So enough said. Sit down and work it!

Men have it the easiest when trying to find the PC muscle. Most of you should be able to feel your PC muscle just behind your testicles and in front of your anus. Yet the best way for anybody to find the PC muscle is by isolating it. One way for women or men to do this is to sit on the toilet and start to urinate. Try to stop the flow of urine midstream by contracting your pelvic-floor muscles. You may want to try using a series of flicks, briefly contracting and releasing the muscles.

If that doesn't work, try pushing down with your pelvic area as though you are having a bowel movement. By repeating this action several times, you will become familiar with the feel of contracting the correct group of muscles. Try not to contract your abdominal, thigh, or buttocks muscles while performing the exercises. Just concentrate on the pelvic area. (Men may experience a slight stinging sensation when they first practice this exercise.)

Another aid to identifying the correct muscle group is to insert your finger into the vagina (in women) or rectum (in men). Try to tighten the muscles, as if holding back urine, around your finger. Do this while the abdominal and thigh muscles remain relaxed.

Women may also strengthen the PC muscle by using a **vaginal cone**, a weighted device that is inserted into the vagina, which can be found at a sex shop. The goal with this apparatus is to try to hold the device in place by contracting the pelvic-floor muscles around it.

Doing Kegel Exercises

Now that you've found the PC muscle, you're anxious to get started on this new exercise routine. The great thing about these exercises is that they can be performed any time and any place. While most people prefer to perform the exercises while lying down or sitting in a chair, you could do it while driving, talking on the phone, watching TV, standing in line at the ATM, waiting for an elevator, or reading this book. Plus, any habitual activity, like every time you brush your teeth, can act as a good reminder.

All right, then. Before we begin the Kegel exercises, here are some Y-BO basics about your PC muscle so you know what's going on while you flex: In contracting this soon-to-be-toned muscle during sex, you will be temporarily reducing the flow of blood to your genital area. When you release the muscle, the blood flow to your pelvic region increases, producing greater vaginal lubrication in women and stronger erections in men, plus heightened awareness for both sexes. Excellent. So you can see that a buff PC muscle is quite a sexual enhancer, and squeezing it is yet another way to eroticize safer sex. No matter how you isolate the PC muscle or which of the following exercises you decide to do, you'll see the same result in bed.

KEGEL EXERCISES FOR WOMEN

Before pursuing the following steps, make sure about a couple of things. The goal of having PC-muscle control is a serious one and you need to set aside some time for yourself to work out, just like you would need to for aerobics or your favorite TV show. Make sure the time for these exercises is a time when you're alone and not likely to be interrupted.

1. Begin by emptying your bladder.
2. Relax and concentrate on contracting just the pelvic-floor muscles.
3. Tighten the pelvic-floor muscles and hold for three counts.
4. Breathe slowly and deeply.
5. Relax the PC muscle completely for three counts.
6. Perform ten exercises of these three counts, three times a day.

Take your time when you're performing these exercises. Don't rush through them. It is not a good idea to increase the number of repetitions and the frequency of exercise to obtain faster results. This doesn't speed up the progress and may cause muscle fatigue and increase your leakage of urine. So take your time with Kegels. As you're doing them, pretend I'm fitness trainer to the stars Kathy Kaehler, talking to you in one of her fitness videos, wearing a sexy thong leotard of course, and we're doing the cool-down. My voice is calm and soothing and we're slow-ly prac-ti-cing the ex-er-cise.

If you can't hold your counts for three seconds, try holding them for just one or two counts until you're able to build up the strength and endurance you need. Gradually, work your way up to ten counts per hold. You can further build your strength and endurance by using resistive devices that help to keep the PC muscle flexed. These may include your finger, a dildo, or vibrator. Simply try to contract the muscle around these.

Another way to achieve greater strength and endurance is to practice short PC muscle flicks, squeezing and releasing them as quickly as you can for a few minutes. Pop in your favorite, upbeat workout music and try to keep up with the beat! You can test your PC muscle by placing one or two of your fingers inside your vagina and imagining that you are starting and stopping your urinary stream. You should notice that the muscles on the sides of the vagina put pressure on your fingers.

KEGEL EXERCISES FOR MEN

Don't think that I forgot about you, men. Everything I just told the ladies holds true for you, too, only your exercises are slightly different. These are important exercises to practice because they're going to help you in the next chapter, when I give you the basics to becoming multi-orgasmic. So without further ado, to strengthen your PC muscle, perform the following steps:

1. Start by holding and releasing your PC muscle fifteen times, twice a day. Do this slowly, concentrating on your prostate, perineum, and anus.

2. Gradually increase the number of squeezes until you're up to seventy-five repetitions, twice a day.

3. Once at seventy-five, you can move on to phase II of the exercise. In phase II, hold your contraction for a count of three instead of releasing immediately, then relax and repeat as many times as you can.

4. Slowly, work up to about fifty of these longer Kegels.

5. Continue these exercises for six weeks, alternating between the longer and shorter Kegels. You should notice results in your orgasms after a month or so.

6. Once you've mastered these exercises, you can squeeze your pelvic-floor muscles when you're having sex, being stimulated, or having an erotic fantasy to make your sexual experience sweeter and more electrifying than ever before.

In general, everyone should notice some improvement in muscle control of this region after four to six weeks, though it may take as long as three months to see and feel a drastic change. Furthermore, all of you can start using your PC muscle as a way to eroticize safer sex. Often an argument against condoms is that they can reduce sensitivity during sex. With PC-muscle control, you control your sex session's sensitivity. Think of all of the sensations you'll experience, and be able to provide your partner, in gripping his condom-covered manhood. Imagine sex that's so good that you'll forget that you're wearing that little latex life preserver over your better-than-ever erection.... Did any of you doubt me?

You're doing Kegel exercises incorrectly if...

✳ You feel discomfort in your abdomen or back while performing these exercises.

✳ You're holding your breath or tightening your chest while trying to contract the pelvic-floor muscles—this could cause you to get a headache when exercising.

Kegel exercises will make you men love her and life as you've never loved them before, plus give you an orgasm intensity previously thought unimaginable. For you ladies, Kegel exercises will turn you into his favorite lusty, love goddess and your vagina into your most valuable asset, plus skyrocket him to best-lover-ever status. Nadia, a 22-year-old sexy, young—and, by the way, eligible—professional boasts about her PC-muscle strength: "PC-muscle squeezes—I'm really good at those. There was this guy I used to sleep with from Austria and I used that muscle with him and he was like, 'Amazing American woman!' because he'd never felt it before. It was really neat to use it because I loved his reaction."

Pressure's on. We have an international reputation to live up to. Do our country proud!

CHAPTER 16

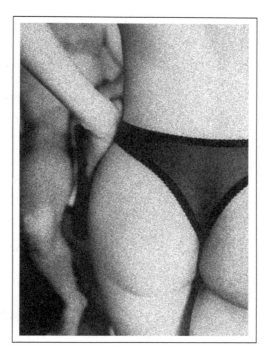

Making a Multi-Orgasmic Man

How can a male become multi-orgasmic?

What are the keys to developing ejaculatory control?

How do you do ejaculatory control exercises?

How can my partner help me out?

The potential to be multi-orgasmic and to have better ejaculatory control is not only exciting for many men, but is thrilling for couples as well. Being multi-orgasmic provides yet another way to eroticize safer sex. Many-a-time, a fellow won't want to wear a condom because he thinks sex feels better without one or because a condom reduces his sensitivity. While the quest for ultimate sensations during sex is certainly a noble one, it's not very knightly to forego condoms and risk contracting or giving an STD or HIV or getting his Guinevere pregnant. The Holy Grail of better, safer, super-sensitive sex is developing ejaculatory control and becoming multi-orgasmic.

By tapping into his multi-orgasmic potential, a guy isn't going to care as much that he has to wear a condom. He'll probably even forget that he's wearing one. Multiple orgasms are that powerful! Besides, wearing a condom actually helps a guy last longer in bed, allowing him to hold off ejaculation longer and to eventually have multiple orgasms. The fact that he can orgasm again and again, partly with a little assistance from his condom, goes way beyond the pleasure of unprotected intercourse.

Everything I'm presenting here on multiple orgasms and ejaculatory control is very quick and basic. Becoming a multi-orgasmic male requires weeks to months of training, lots of patience, and much more knowledge than this chapter presents. If you're serious about exploring your multi-orgasmic potential, I highly recommend getting a book that is completely devoted to it, like Chia and Abrams' *The Multi-Orgasmic Man*.

The tricks and techniques in this chapter should be useful in helping you to postpone orgasm. The central concept in having multiple orgasms is developing ejaculatory control. There are only certain times during arousal when a male can consciously make changes in his behavior to influence when he ejaculates. This "**control zone period**" is from the beginning of penile stimulation to just before the point where ejaculation becomes inevitable. With ejaculatory control, you'll usually have a choice as to when to ejaculate. You can let your arousal rise to a high level and then more or less level off until you want to come. In becoming multi-orgasmic, a man learns to separate his different arousal sensations and postpone ejaculation by reveling in orgasm. This can be done because ejaculating and having an orgasm are not one in the same—they can happen separately.

To Make or Break

Cole expresses the sentiments that many of you males probably feel right now: "I've never had a multiple orgasm and I didn't even realize that men could. I feel like I'm missing out on a whole new world!"

Becoming a multi-orgasmic male requires the ability to develop your sexual strength and sensitivity. It involves both physical and mental practice and an awareness of how your body operates when it's sexually aroused. To reach a basic understanding of what happens to your body when you're sexually excited and when you're about to ejaculate, we should probably put you in the right context and get you aroused. So grab your copy of *Hustler,* drop your pants, and... just kidding. We don't need to go that far. All I need for you to do is to pretend that you're masturbating. Get in the mood like you normally would. I'll even set the scene for you....

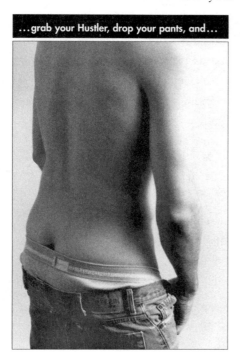

...grab your Hustler, drop your pants, and...

Pretend that you're at a dance club and your dream girl comes up to you in a tight, slightly see-through tank top and one of the shortest miniskirts you've ever seen. You're practically panting, your eyes bulging out of your head, as the two of you start talking. She says that she'd love to "have" you and wants to give you her phone number. As she's about to write it down, she clumsily "drops" her pen. She gives you her most vixen smile before bending over to pick it up. Wouldn't you know it, she doesn't have any underwear on....

I'll let you finish that one. Remember, this is still pretend, so don't go off and get too excited on me. We need to see this visualization through.

All right then, you're getting aroused and getting an erection and passing through the excitement phase of your sexual response cycle. The next part is where it all starts to get a bit tricky: You enter the cycle's **contractile** or **emission phase**. Here, as your prostate contracts and empties your semen into your urethra, you must make a pretty weighty decision: Are you going to continue doing whatever you're doing and enjoy the immediate gratification of ejaculation? Or should you maybe slow down your pace a bit, postpone ultimate fulfillment, and end with the grand finale of multiple orgasms? If you do choose to come, you enter the **expulsion phase**, during which your semen shoots down your urethra and out of your penis.

If you choose to hold off, you'll stay in the contractile phase and will feel a series of mild or intense prostate contractions lasting three to five seconds. These are pelvic orgasms or "**contractile-phase orgasms**." When you feel these contractions, you need to decide again if you're going to continue to the point of no return or momentarily decrease stimulation long enough to gain control over your state of arousal. This may be hard to do since the fluttering sensation your prostate is producing feels so good that it makes you want to let go.

If you continue to hold off, aspiring for multiple orgasms, you want to try to stay as close as possible to ejaculatory inevitability, reveling in the contractile-phase orgasms, without reaching ejaculation. At this stage, you'll feel pleasure and the release of prostate contractions, PC-muscle contractions, and anal-sphincter contractions. Here, to postpone ejaculation, you need to do all of the following:

* Squeeze the PC muscle around your prostate. This will help you to maintain some control over these spine-tingling spasms and develop better pelvis sensitivity.

* Push with your finger on your **million-dollar point**, the indentation on your perineum just in front of your anus, while contract-

ing your PC muscle. Doing this when you're about to ejaculate can help to stop the ejaculatory reflex. Furthermore, pushing on this spot can force more blood into your penis, making it throb quite nicely. This area is best stimulated only after you're fully aroused and erect.

* Draw energy away from your genitals and up your spine. (This requires a lot of mind work that you need to practice for quite some time.) This relieves some of the pressure on the genitals and your urge to ejaculate. Your arousal may waver a bit as you prepare for the next orgasm.

* Practice ejaculatory-control exercises (see the following section).

Note: You may have to stop arousal entirely before reaching the contractile phase if you're prone to ejaculating. There is a chance that you will ejaculate as you practice this. Don't get frustrated or disappointed if this happens; just keep at it.

Ejaculatory Control Development

As was said earlier, developing ejaculatory control can help a man develop an awareness of his various arousal sensations and recognize when he might be nearing ejaculatory inevitability. Ejaculatory control helps him to hold off until he wants to expel semen.

Better ejaculatory control means longer, and usually more enjoyable, sex. Men who have achieved such control feel much more confident and better about themselves as lovers, and their partners usually don't complain about this talent either. If you can develop ejaculatory control, you can enjoy high levels of sexual arousal without coming right away. Men who gain control over their ejaculations report that their orgasms feel better, "fuller," or "more complete" than they had been previously.

SEVEN KEYS TO DEVELOPING EJACULATORY CONTROL

There are seven main components involved in ejaculatory control, and there are ejaculatory control exercises to help you develop these. All of the exercises must be practiced solo before they are done with a partner. If you keep these keys in mind, you may experience multiple orgasms in as little as one to two weeks. You will also master the ejaculatory control techniques in anywhere from three to six months.

1. **Learn to breathe properly.** Panting, choppy grunts and holding your breath aren't going to cut it. Take a few deep breaths to help ease the arousal and tension that can lead to your cumming quickly. Breathe deeply into the bottom of your lungs, through your nose—*belly breathing*. Holding your breath for several moments until your urge to orgasm subsides is necessary for you to be able to stop yourself from ejaculating, plus it helps you to expand that feeling of orgasm throughout your body.

2. It's all about strength, **mind strength**, that is. Concentration is key. Start with a simple mind exercise by counting to 100 without letting your mind wander. Sound pretty silly and easy? Try making each count worth one exhale and inhale. This slows the pace of your counting dramatically, unless you like to hyperventilate when you breathe, and becomes difficult because of the concentration it requires for you to solely focus on the breathing.

3. You have to be able **to attend more fully to your own sensations of arousal and tension** when you, or your partner, are stimulating your penis. Learn to be aware of your arousal level. This will help you monitor when you'll need to slow down stimulation to prevent ejaculation. As your penis is being stroked, you need to focus your attention on your penis or scrotum, especially the places where you can feel increases in fullness, tingling, or other arousing sensations.

4. **Use mental power and visual imagery** as much as possible whenever you find yourself haunted by that unavoidable, occasional thought: "Chad, you come too fast." Challenge that idea! Argue with it and change it. As soon as you've gotten a grip on that debilitating thought, imagine yourself having long-lasting intercourse with good control. This type of visual imagery can be really fun because you can exercise the power of your fantasizing abilities as well. For example, imagine entering her—her warmth,

her wetness, her grip, and you're just, oh god...that's right, feeling relaxed and comfortable. Feel the sensation of just being still inside of her—no movement—for a moment or so. The Apollo has landed and it feels *so good*. Enjoy it!

Then imagine slow movements. You're still taking it easy, still enjoying the feeling of being inside of her, still in control. Then, gradually increase the pace of your thrusts. On occasion, visualize that you're slowing down. Each time you imagine yourself thrusting, *gradually* increase the pace of your thrusts until you're calmly and easily moving almost as much as you want.

Now see yourself in the saddle. You're moving hard. You're in control. Who's your daddy?! You're about to come! Now imagine yourself slowing down and stopping *all* movement. Just stop thrusting and experience the pleasure. Ahhhh.... Then gradually increase the movements again, slowly building up until you're letting your body do what it wants. This time, whenever you want, imagine an explosive ejaculation.

Such mental exercises will help you prepare for the actual physical exercises. You may have to rehearse them over and over again. Furthermore, you'll need to spend a few seconds rehearsing for these physical exercises by visualizing yourself doing them perfectly before moving on to the real thing.

5. **Know what to do during a stop!** During a stop, you can simply relax and enjoy the pleasant feelings of decreasing arousal or you can talk briefly to your partner if she's around, like, "So how about that Penn State football team? Kicked butt Saturday...." Try to really experience the control you're exercising over your ejaculatory process and take several deep breaths to help yourself relax. If you have the urge to come during a stop, you can squeeze your penis by placing your first two fingers on the underside of your penis and your thumb on top, or by pulling your scrotal sac down.

6. **Adapt to your state of arousal.** You need to be able to make changes in your behavior that will prevent or delay ejaculation, like either stopping completely or doing something else, such as taking the time to stimulate your nipples instead of your genitals to maintain ejaculatory control. This key actually goes hand in hand with attending to your arousal. The goal is to stop stimulation anytime you're in the control zone, not when you're just about to reach the point of inevitability. Think of your orgasm as a sneeze and remember the occasions you've tried to suppress that big "Ah choo!" When you do stop, do so for different lengths of time, anywhere from ten seconds to a minute and a half. See what works best for you.

7. **Strengthen your PC muscle.** First, find out where it is (see Chapter 15 for help with this one). Feel it through your perineum (behind your testes and in front of your anus). Since orgasm builds from your prostate, and your pelvic muscles surround your prostate, you'll want to learn to squeeze this muscle around your prostate to control your ejaculation.

EXERCISES FOR EJACULATORY CONTROL

The following are masturbation and "with a partner" exercises that should be performed two to three times per week, or even daily. Committing to such an "exercise regime" should eventually result in ejaculatory control, one of the key components in tapping into your multi-orgasmic potential.

Ejaculatory control exercises can also help those suffering from premature ejaculation, a sexual difficulty that causes men to ejaculate more quickly than they would like.

Note: It is crucial that you do not force erection during any of the following exercises:

Masturbation Exercises (fifteen minutes)

Solo Exercise

The goal of this exercise is to masturbate for fifteen minutes without ejaculating.

1. With a dry hand, focus on your pelvic area or penis. Be aware of how aroused and tense you are. While this can be an arousing activity, try to stay relaxed.

2. When you feel that you are in the control zone, that "not quite about to come, but it's just a couple of thrusts away feeling," stop all stimulation and tune into the sensations you're feeling. Take a few deep breaths.

3. When your arousal and tension levels have greatly dropped (this could take anywhere from ten seconds to more than one minute), resume stimulation.

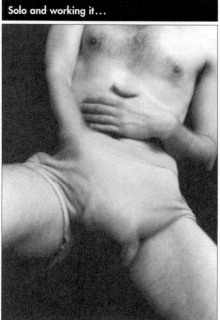

Solo and working it...

4. Repeat the steps, only this time use a lubricant or massage oil on your hand. When you need only one or two stimulation stops over the course of a fifteen-minute session, you're ready to move on to the next solo exercise.

Solo and Working It

The goal of this exercise is to masturbate for fifteen minutes without ejaculating and without stopping.

1. Once your arousal and tension levels are in the control zone, change your stimulation technique in order to control your ejaculatory process. Changes may include slowing down the pace, changing the site of maximum stimulation (like focusing on your shaft versus the head), and changing the type of stroke (e.g., using circular instead of long strokes). Try one change at a time, testing which one works best for you.

2. Repeat the steps, this time using lubricant on your hand. Once you're comfortable masturbating for fifteen minutes using this method and are using only subtle adjustments, you can move on to "with a partner" ejaculatory control exercises.

"With a Partner" Exercises

Before starting the following partner exercises, be sure to talk to your lover about the various techniques and what is expected of each of you in order for these exercises to work. Figure out a word that you will use—your "signal word"—to signal when your lover should stop and start stimulation. Make sure that both of you are relaxed and comfortable before starting an exercise, and that you'll be comfortable in your chosen positions for the next fifteen minutes of the exercise. Also, before you advance to each exercise, make sure that you need no more than two stops during a fifteen-minute period and that you feel confident of your control. Take your time advancing through the exercises. There's no rush!

During each exercise, keep your focus on your arousal and tension levels, not on your partner. She may turn you on so much that thinking too much about her aching for you, putting the condom on you, pulling you into her, and murmuring to do her could blow it all in just a matter of seconds. Make sure your partner understands the exercises and the role you need her to play in order to help you.

Before you practice each of these exercises, grab a condom. Using a condom during these exercises is not only a good idea because of pregnancy, STD, and HIV prevention, but because a condom can help you maintain an erection and postpone ejaculation. As you practice these exercises, you're going to really appreciate this extra assistance from your rubber!

Work Your Penis

1. With her unlubricated hand, your partner stimulates your penis in ways that arouse you. If necessary, give her pointers on how to stroke you.

2. When your arousal and tension levels need to be decreased, tell her to stop. This is where a signal word comes in handy.

3. As soon as the levels have fallen, let her know that she can resume stimulation.

4. When ready, repeat these steps, this time with your partner now using a lubricant, oil, or lotion on her hand.

Work It a Little Bit More

1. Repeat the steps from the "Work Your Penis" exercise, only, as your partner stimulates your penis with a dry hand, you will delay ejaculation by telling her to slow down the pace or change the stroking technique, instead of stopping.

2. Repeat the techniques you were just using, except now she will use a lubricant on her hand.

3. (optional step) Repeat the above, only she can use her mouth instead of her hand.

Tease Your Penis

1. Lie on your back and have her sit on your thighs.

2. Once erect, rub your penis gently for a few seconds on her inner thighs and enjoy the sensation that is produced.

3. Remember to take deep, relaxing breaths before starting the next and subsequent steps.

4. Take a few seconds' rest, then do the same thing in her pubic hair.

5. Take another quick rest.

6. Now rub your penis on the outer lips of her vagina and enjoy the experience.

7. Pause, and then put the head of your penis between her vaginal lips and enjoy that for a moment.

8. Repeat the exercise until you are able to do it without anxiety and without the urge to ejaculate.

9. Once you can comfortably go through the whole exercise, do it again, only this time let her hand guide your penis.

Gradual Insertion (five minutes)

1. One of you should place your erect penis just at the opening of her vagina.

2. Take a few seconds to get used to having it there.

3. Once comfortable, move the penis into the vagina a tad, about an inch.

4. Take a few seconds to get used to just having it there.

5. Continue doing this until your entire penis is inside her. Move slowly, staying aware of what is happening to you.

6. Then stay that way for a few minutes and focus on your arousal and tension.

7. Feel how it is to have your penis surrounded by her vagina—the temperature, the moisture, the texture.

8. If at any time you think you're about to lose control, slow your breathing with some deep breaths.

Note: Both of you have to realize that this is not intercourse and that she needs to stay pretty still during these exercises. The whole purpose of doing all of this is for you to feel greater comfort in simply being inside of her. Your lover might get a little frustrated that these exercises seem to totally tease her. Make sure that you don't leave her hanging when you finish a practice session. Please her to no end. Furthermore, make sure the two of you are having fun on this sexual adventure. Don't be afraid to laugh—have a sense of humor about it. This will make things much easier.

It's in There (fifteen minutes)

1. This is a continuation of the previous exercise, with the goal being to have your penis in her vagina with little or no movement. Once again, she needs to be still.

2. Either of you can slowly insert your penis.

3. Once fully inside, just be there—for fifteen minutes.

4. During that time, you may find yourself losing your erection. If so, ask her to contract her pelvic muscles a few times, or you can move slightly, just enough to keep it hard.

Pick Up the Pace

1. Decide on a sexual position. This will determine who will be doing the moving—the slow thrusting—for this exercise.

2. The thrusting partner should start with a very slow pace and allow you to get comfortable with it before increasing movement.

3. After a while, make thrusting a little faster, while you take some deep breaths.

4. When you feel that you can handle that speed without losing control, increase the speed again.

5. Continue this until the active partner is moving at a fairly steady pace, though not full-blown thrusting. If she's the one in control, make sure that she doesn't start thrusting to satisfy herself.

6. Repeat these steps, only with the other partner doing the moving—maybe in a different position.

7. Once steps 1–6 are completed, repeat them, only with both of you moving. Practice as much as you'd like until both of you are able to move comfortably and be in control, getting as fast as your heart desires!

Every man has the ability to develop his ejaculatory control and every man has the potential to be multi-orgasmic, though not every male will be able to experience having more than one orgasm. While these exercises may be helpful in mastering ejaculatory control and discovering your multi-orgasmic potential, you need to experiment with your own combination of techniques and positions to find out what works for you. Miguel tells of an ejaculatory control trick, not mentioned in this chapter, that works for him: "I usually have good ejaculatory control when I'm trying really hard to keep going. Flexing my ass helps in being able to thrust a little longer. You just let go of your muscles when you get close to ejaculating and the urge to ejaculate lets off."

So try practicing these exercises in different positions and try different tricks of your own. With each new one, you will have to work on your control, but just start out slowly, gradually increasing the tempo. Slowly, your partner can pick up the pace too, until both of you can move and relish in it, knowing that you have total ejaculatory control.

Before signing out from this chapter, I need to stress that developing ejaculatory control and becoming multi-orgasmic do not happen overnight. In a world of fast food, the Internet, and instant pudding, it can be really hard to be patient. I, for one, am all about immediate gratification in life, so I can empathize with your desire to master ejaculatory control A.S.A.P. Just remember, in exercising your ejaculatory control and discovering your multi-orgasmic potential, good things come (and many times) to those who wait.

RESOURCES

Mantak Chia and Douglas Abrams' *The Multi-Orgasmic Man*

Barbara Keesling's *Sexual Pleasure* and *Sexual Healing* (www.hunterhouse.com)

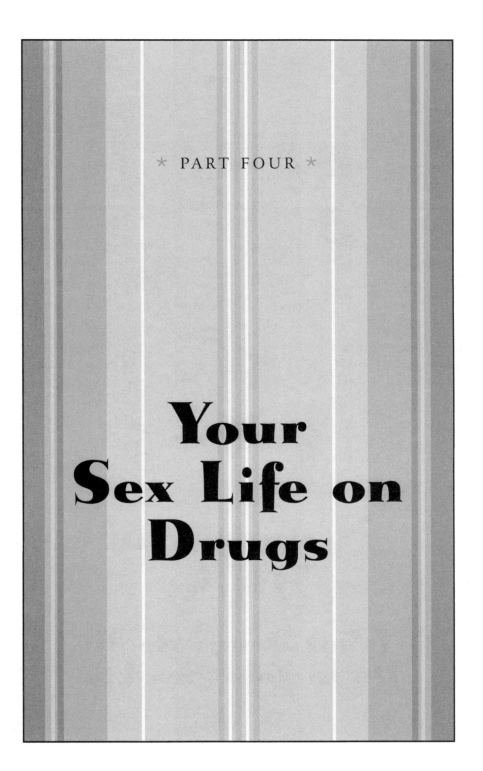

* PART FOUR *

Your
Sex Life on
Drugs

CHAPTER 17

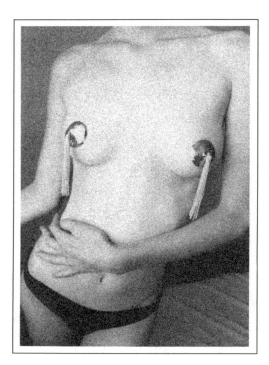

Horny and High:

What Drugs Really Do to Your Sex Life

Do drugs make for better sex?

What are the side effects of stimulants?

What are the dangers of combining sex and drugs?

Sex and Drugs

So you're thinking about alternative ways to enhance your sex life. Or you've heard that combining sex and drugs is absolutely out of this world and something you *have* to try sometime. Or you've simply wondered on occasion what would *really* happen if you smoked up, snorted, or shot up a drug before a sexual experience.

Does the drug truly make sex that much better? Or does the person merely think that sex is better because he's using a drug? Or is it that she doesn't remember a single thing that was going on while she was high, so it must have been a really good time?

With this chapter, I'm not advocating drug use. I matter-of-factly want you to know the real scoop as to what a drug can do to you, or for you, and your sex life. I'm going to dispel some myths circulating about drugs and sex. I'm laying it all out so that you'll be better informed as to the true consequences of sex and drugs.

While almost any drug can seem to have a certain amount of appeal as far as the high it offers, there are always at least a few negative, and possibly deadly, side effects that should make you think twice before using any of these substances. Furthermore, you should be wary of mixing sex and drugs since this combination more often than not makes you forget all about practicing safer sex, and that's not erotic. Sex while high on a drug increases your chance of acquiring an STD or HIV or getting pregnant—definitely good reasons to stay away from these substances, especially if you're out for a little worry-free somp'in, somp'in.

> Nicotine, the drug found in tobacco that cigarette smokers become addicted to, has been found to be more prevalent among impotent men. This is because nicotine constricts blood vessels and thus there's less blood being pumped to the penis to fill an erection. Think about that the next time you see a dude light up at a bar.

Marijuana

Cannabis, hashish, grass, hemp, pot, reefer, weed . . . no matter what the term, we've all heard of this drug before. Nearly as plentiful as its nicknames are the number of ways humans have learned to use it. We inhale it from a bong, smoke it from a rolled joint or a packed pipe, or cook or bake it in foods, like brownies, to eat.

Marijuana is a drug that distorts your perception of reality—increasing your heart rate, lowering your blood pressure, and limiting your control of movement. It is an attractive drug because of the feelings of contentment and relaxation it produces and because it may be accompanied by a loss of inhibition, bouts of laughter, continuous talking, increased sensitivity to audio and visual effects, and an increased sensitivity to touch, smell, taste, and movement.

Users report that pot acts as a stimulant, with more than 60 percent of them claiming that it enhances sex. This claim is partly based on pot producing the sensation that time is being stretched out, thus prolonging and intensifying sensations, including sexual sensations.

There is no scientific documentation of marijuana's effects as an aphrodisiac.

Theo, a 27-year-old graduate student, is among the 60 percent who hail the positives of sex when stoned:

I have never had a bad experience when stoned. In fact, the best sex I ever had was when my girlfriend and I went camping and smoked a joint before having sex. Sharing the high made us feel more attached to each other. As we started hooking up, everything was spinning— your brain goes so fast when you're going at it stoned. At the same time, I was having this great rush. I felt so safe and warm in that little tent with her.

Yet while Theo loves getting stoned and making love, he does warn that sex while high should only be done on occasion: "If you do it on a regular basis, it doesn't make the times you do it as great or as special. Plus, some argue that marijuana is a 'gateway drug' and I don't want to do it too much for fear I'll move on to harder drugs for the same high."

While for some users, like Theo, marijuana can be a stimulant, there are times when it can be an anti-motivational drug, which is why the drug is also classified as a sedative-hypnotic. Sex while high may cause you to lose interest, lose focus, lose your feelings of arousal, as well as make you very tired and paranoid—states of mind and body that aren't appealing whatsoever.

Furthermore, one of the short-term effects of weed is that it reduces your ability to perform tasks requiring concentration and coordination, like stimulating her clitoris with your fingers to bring her to orgasm as you do her doggie-style. Stoned sex can be very unfulfilling, frustrating, and sloppy.

Kirsten, as a junior in college, felt such debilitating effects from smoking pot before sex one night:

> Mark and I had both had a long day and a joint seemed like the perfect way to start the night. Only, once we were stoned, it was so hard to get motivated to have sex. Neither of us wanted to be the one doing all of the work—all of the thrusting. So the whole time we were having sex, we kept rolling over, playfully arguing and laughing, "No, you on top!" "No, you on top!" It was pretty funny, but turned me off to combining sex and pot for a while. I couldn't understand all of the hype about it.

It's just as well that Kirsten's experience ended up like it did. Pot use can cause confusion, disorientation, recent memory loss, lack of balance and stability, loss of muscle strength, vaginal dryness, and tremors, while anxiety and paranoia may occur with higher doses.

Longer-term use can lead to asthma, bronchitis, damage to the respiratory system and tissue, reddening of the eyes, *changes in your sex drive,* and *infertility. Your sex drive becomes diminished, if not completely extinguished, over time.* For men, one of the long-term effects of heavy pot use is a *decrease* in testosterone levels, which can cause infertility. For women, one of the long-term effects of heavy marijuana use is an *increase* in testosterone levels, which can also cause infertility.

Ecstasy

Known as a "jewel of a drug," "love drug," and "hug drug," Ecstasy is the hallucinogenic compound MDMA, which is in the amphetamine family. It is usually taken in pill form but can be snorted, smoked, or injected as well. It can provoke intense, energetic, spiritual highs and euphoria or lead to warm, loving relaxation and sensual enhancement. It's popular among late-night dance-club- and rave-goers. People on "E," or "X," say that they connect freely and openly with each other and help each other promote deep inner thinking and analysis. Music sounds better; people look hotter. Users report that E does not make them necessarily feel sexual, but sensual, beautiful, and sometimes dangerous.

Ecstasy is the kind of euphoric drug that gives you what you put into it, thus covering a wide range of human emotions, experiences, and passions. It increases feelings of empathy and understanding. Ireland, a 23-year-old rave-goer and student, explains this E-experience:

> E is great for women because it's touchy, feely—caressing. Women like that. You know, indirect stimulation is better than direct. What makes E even nicer is that it's usually done in a public place so that people are complimenting each other more. There's more flattery and kind gestures. It's such a euphoric drug! It makes you feel pretty, desirable, satisfied. . . .
> It gets rid of your insecurities.

Studies on young women who take drugs recreationally while raving have found that sex is *not* one of the foremost pleasures offered by Ecstasy. At raves, dancers are more motivated to concentrate on the pleasures of dancing—the sensations of the body, mind, and soul—than on sex. Thus, many people are attracted to E and raves, as opposed to an alcohol-based nightlife, because they enjoy the group setting, one where the pressure to have sex and the emphasis on sex have been removed. Sex is usually the last thing on a person's mind at a rave.

Sexual safety is an attraction of E and raves for young women; women sometimes enjoy kissing men at raves because it feels good and safe since it is not going to involve sex. Most women at raves say that they do not have casual sex on the nights they rave. For the handful who are into sex after an E trip, the drug is said to be ideal in that it produces "long, slow sex" when done with some marijuana. This is probably because of pot's debilitating effects.

Like women, men on E are also less interested in sex and do not expect sex. Most men have the opposite of an erection—a *shrinking penis*, which may be one of the reasons guys don't focus nearly as much on sex as they normally would, and one good reason why this is not a very attractive drug.

Luigi, while in the Navy as a teenager, had on occasion done Ecstasy while raving:

> Being on E reduces your inhibitions. You do things you normally would
> never do, like give your girlfriend a full-body massage. At raves, every-
> body enjoys each other's company, and they touch each other all over
> without feeling threatened in any way. The key element of E is that it is
> a sensual versus a sexual drug; it enhances your sensory perception.
> Sex is less of a focus.

The effects of E kick in within thirty minutes, and last four to six hours. Aftereffects can last for days to weeks. Coming down from E, people often report feelings of loneliness, coupled with a still-enhanced sense of touch. It is at this point that safer-sex plans can be forgotten. Other drawbacks to using E are a variety of physical symptoms, like jaw-clenching, teeth-grinding, eye wiggles, tightened muscles, sweating, chills, auditory effects, nausea, shaking, next-day sleepiness, and increased heart rate, blood pressure, and body temperature. If a user has been dancing a lot, his/her temperature goes up and there's a great deal of water loss, possibly resulting in dehydration and hypothermia. In extreme cases, this has proved fatal.

Some people experience a brief depression the next day and with repeated use can suffer from enduring depression and anxiety. On occasion in people with asthma, heart conditions, diabetes, epilepsy, psychosis, or depression, toxic reactions can result. A hit of "X," or "E," taken with anti-depressants, migraine medications, decongestants, diet pills, or amphetamines can even trigger a sudden, life-threatening stroke! So like I said, all of these drugs have some negative side effects that your body might be better off without.

Ecstasy users try to avoid such negative symptoms and consequences by drinking lots of water to replenish body fluids, avoiding alcohol, and taking moments to stop moving, to breathe deeply, and to relax. It is one of the few drugs where users actually agree that "less is more."

Poppers

Poppers is a term for amyl, butyl, or isobutyl nitrate that opens up the blood vessels, making the blood rush to your brain, causing a very quick, short high. It produces heightened sensations during orgasm, probably by dilating blood vessels in the genitals. This drug is sometimes used by people when having anal sex because it relaxes the sphincter muscle tissue of the anus.

While such a relaxing effect can make sex more pleasurable, it may cause users to be unaware of painful tearing and bleeding that may be a sign that sexual activity should slow down or stop. Hence, the drug is strongly associated with HIV transmission among people practicing anal intercourse. Many users find that as soon as they are comfortable with their body's limits and know how to relax before anal sex, poppers become unnecessary. Plus, popper-free sex can help avoid the dizziness, headaches, fainting, and nervous-system damage that can be highly undesirable side effects of this drug.

Cocaine

Considered the drug of choice for enhancing sexual experiences, cocaine is a powerful, central nervous system stimulant that heightens alertness, inhibits appetite and the need for sleep, and provides intense feelings of pleasure. Used for its potent euphoric and energizing effects, its users can *quickly* become dependent. Cocaine in its powder form is usually snorted into the nostrils, though it may also be rubbed onto the mucous lining of the mouth, rectum, or vagina. To experience its effects more quickly and to heighten their intensity, users may inject it, thus increasing the risk of getting HIV or hepatitis from unsterile needles.

The short-term effects of cocaine include making some users feel talkative, invincible, and mentally alert, especially to sight, sound, and touch, while others may feel anxious, panic-stricken, or contemplative. Some people find that cocaine allows them to perform simple intellectual and physical tasks more quickly; others experience the exact opposite effect.

Some persons on cocaine report that the drug increases their sexual feelings when they first start using it. The stimulant makes them feel alert, sexy, and confident, although sometimes also a little paranoid. The highs this drug offers, however, such as increased sexual desire, enhanced sensuality, and delayed orgasm, are fairly short-lived. The cocaine boost one experiences is actually illusory, all in the brain.

Furthermore, as coke use continues, the reverse effects are felt, with users reporting a *loss* of interest in sexual activity and desire, *orgasm disorders,* and *erectile disorders.* Shirl-dog explains his body's biggest reaction to the drug: "Sex while on coke makes my penis go limp." Enough said.

Another aspect of mixing sex and cocaine is that the drug is associated with high-risk sexual behavior in men and women. People who combine sex and crack (a form of cocaine) are more than 50 percent more likely to have a sexually transmitted infection, such as gonorrhea, than crack users who do not use crack during sex. It's possible that the feelings of invincibility that crack creates allow users to deny the need for condoms. Users also tend to have more sex partners in a year and are less likely to use condoms.

Besides the negative effects the drug can have on your sex life, using larger amounts of cocaine to intensify your "high" can also lead to bizarre, erratic, and violent behavior. Such effects include vertigo (the feeling that your surroundings are whirling about sickeningly), paranoia, nausea, blurred vision, fever, muscle spasms, *erectile failure,* chest pain, and coma. An overdose can lead to death.

Over time, the user no longer experiences euphoria and instead feels restlessness, extreme excitability, insomnia, hallucinations, and delusions. Ultimately, a heavy user may also suffer from mood swings, *loss of interest in sex,* and weight loss. Additionally, coke use causes *abnormalities in sperm production.* If you have any concerns whatsoever about your future offspring's welfare, consider that well before you pick up this drug habit.

Crystal

Crystal meth (speed) is an amphetamine that increases your breathing and heart rate, raises your blood pressure, and can cause dehydration. Eaten, injected, or smoked, a high can last up to two whole days. While the "rush" of sex sessions is enhanced, the chemical can make it *difficult for men to obtain or maintain an erection.* For both sexes, use over time affects users' sex drive, in that speed causes problems like anxiety, depression, and fatigue—emotional states that affect your libido.

There is also increased risk of skin damage and split condoms during sex on speed, since your body is less sensitive. Thus, the chances of HIV transmission also increase. In addition, crystal holds back alcohol's intoxicating effects, so you may drink to excess without realizing it and end up doing something that is harmful to your health, or deadly.

Heroin

Heroin is a highly addictive drug derived from morphine, which comes from the opium poppy. It affects the brain's pleasure systems and interferes with the brain's ability to perceive pain. It is a fast-acting, psychologically and physically addictive drug that reaches the brain in fifteen to thirty seconds if injected into a vein and in seven seconds if smoked.

The high from heroin is experienced as intense pleasure, an "orgasmic rush," followed by peacefulness, lack of pain, and euphoria. Many people are attracted to the drug because the high is said to be better than sex, better than any orgasm ever attained from sex. Psychologically, users might think so, but physiologically their bodies are a dead "no-go" when it comes to sex.

The user's euphoric state soon becomes one of drowsiness, inactivity, the inability to concentrate, nodding off, small pupils, droopy eyelids, limited vision, slowed breathing or respiratory depression, nausea and vomiting, lack of appetite, constipation, increased urination, itching or burning on the skin, low body temperature, irregular blood pressure and heart rate, menstrual irregularity, and sweating.

As far as sex goes, the effects of this drug on your body result in *reduced sex drive, decreased sexual pleasure,* and even *indifference to sex.* This drug has a *strong suppressive effect on sexual desire and response, inhibits orgasm,* and *produces erectile dysfunction* and *retarded ejaculation.* Long-term use of heroin leads to *decreased testosterone levels* in men. For those who find all of that appealing, remember that as a tolerance develops, more and more of the drug is needed to get the same effect, which also eats a huge chunk out of your wallet.

This is a drug not to be fooled with. Any dose can be unusually potent, leading to overdose, coma, and possible death. Unsterile equipment can be contaminated and dirty needles may transmit HIV and hepatitis. Physical withdrawal is grueling, including symptoms like vomiting, nausea, diarrhea, cramping, and severe shaking. It can take months or even years to recover from the physical addiction; the psychological addiction is a life-long battle.

Drugs like the ones I've described can cloud your judgment, making it harder for you to know right from wrong, and distract you from reality. Drugs can make you do things you may wish you never had done, like making a fool out of yourself, having unplanned sex, having sex without thinking about the consequences, and forgetting to use a condom. Drugs also make you believe that you're having more fun than you really are. Seems like the majority of people out there are very aware of this, with studies showing that few people use drugs before sex.

I would hope that you have enough respect for yourself and your health to realize that drugs aren't the way to go in dealing with or enhancing anything in life, especially your sexual experiences. The best kind of sex involves you having control over your body, you getting things going, and you being safe. That's erotic, not some drug. Plus, who wants to be with a partner who needs a drug for a good time in the sack? Bit of an insult to present company if a partner is always high or tripping, if you know what I mean.

RESOURCES

For more information on drugs, visit:

Dance Safe Organization: www.dancesafe.org

National Institute on Drug Abuse: www.nida.nih.gov

CHAPTER 18

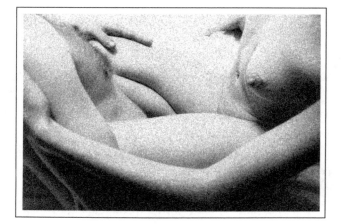

Why Don't We Get Drunk and Screw?

Is alcohol an aphrodisiac?

How does alcohol affect me?

What are the risks involved in drinking and sex?

What are date-rape drugs?

How can I reduce my risk of being drugged and sexually assaulted?

Alcohol has long been considered an aphrodisiac. The strong link between sex and alcohol, which dates back to ancient times, is so strong that societies today still believe in the power of alcohol to induce and enhance sexual pleasure. Liquor equals libido, lust, and love. What better equation is there than that? Best yet, liquor doesn't always equal liable. Part of alcohol's popularity is that our culture often portrays the state of drunkenness as a temporary form of insanity, where you and your sexual behaviors can run rampant without fear that you've done wrong: "I wouldn't have slept with your girlfriend, buddy, if I hadn't been so drunk—honest!"

When drinking, most people conveniently attribute responsibility for their actions to their state of intoxication rather than to themselves. This makes being intoxicated a great pastime for when you want to do all those things you wouldn't dare do sober, like urinate in public; have sex with multiple partners while on spring break; or make a stumbling, slobbering fool of yourself while out on the town.

Alcohol is a big part of our culture and how we conduct ourselves socially. It's available at almost any kind of social event, promoting a certain festive atmosphere in which people can loosen up, be "themselves," and *even* dare to be sexual. "Come here, baby, I'm feeling so sexy right now with this beer breath." We're socialized to believe that if we're drinking, then we're having a great time. "No sibiously, Ine fine. Dis was da best pardy ebba. I dust need a libble more time with de poor-porcelain god here—no wait—yeah here. Hiachhhh!!!…"

About two in three women and nearly one in two men believe that alcohol enhances sexual pleasure. They're not too far off, since alcohol *in small amounts* can increase one's libido, decrease sexual inhibitions, and add to the fun. Yet people often drink much more than small amounts, and that's when we hear all of those stories about alcohol taking away from one's sexual performance, leading to undesirable consequences, and not mixing so well with sex. You have to wonder what it really does to our bodies. So what's the scoop? Is alcohol truly an aphrodisiac?

Alcohol and Expectations

Expectations play a huge role in sexual arousal. When people drink, they expect a certain outcome, and thus they tend to act in ways that enhance the likelihood that the outcome will occur. "I bet that with a few drinks in my system I could totally hit on that bodacious babe at this year's holiday work party. I'm all over those martinis, then all over her!"

Quite the social lubricant, alcohol is seen as an aphrodisiac because it helps people relax, reduces their social anxiety, and helps boost their self-confidence. Studies have found that women tend to drink to enhance their sociability and men drink to experience more aggressiveness and arousal, including sexual arousal, and to express socially inappropriate behavior.

Yvonne on a Soapbox

It is mostly because we have these "alcohol expectations" that I decided to devote an entire chapter to alcohol and sex. Young adults love these myths about alcohol because the myths let them get away with some really stupid things.

Since there are so many misconceptions about alcohol as an aphrodisiac, about what it does to our bodies, and how it makes us so sexual, I want you to know the real skinny on it all. I'm tired of hearing people's stories about sex *while they were drunk*, or how they were only able to hook up with so and so *because they were drunk*, or how they wouldn't have done something sexual *if they hadn't been so drunk*. I'm sick of people blaming alcohol for many of their sexual adventures and decisions, using it as an excuse for those times they were seemingly sex-crazed.

I want people to be more responsible for what they do and say when they're buzzed or intoxicated. I want them to accept that they're as accountable for their words and deeds drunk as sober. I want people to stop blaming the alcohol. I want people to quit coming up with excuses for the stuff they do when they're loaded. I want for people to feel that they can be sexual *without* the alcohol.

The Real Deal on Alcohol and Sex

Because of the widely held cultural belief that alcohol is an aphrodisiac, many young people think that alcohol is a "cure" for their sexual inadequacies, insecurities, and dysfunctions. People who strongly believe that alcohol has a significant effect on their sexual arousal are usually people who also have high levels of sexual guilt. People with high expectations about alcohol use and negative attitudes toward sex are more likely to drink in sexual situations.

Notice I keep saying "beliefs"? The "disinhibiting" effects of alcohol are all in your head, with your brain operating very much on an "if-then" line of thinking: "*If* I drink, *then* I'll work up the nerve to hit on that guy" or "*If* I drink, *then* I'm not responsible for leading her on."

Research has shown that subjects who *believe* that they have consumed alcohol, even though they really have not, show increased levels of sociability, aggression, and sexuality. In both sexes, greater sexual arousal has been indicated by individuals who thought they had received alcoholic beverages, regardless of the actual alcohol content. What all of this means is that the *belief* that you're drinking alcohol is more influential in determining your behavior than the actual kind of beverage or amount of alcohol you're consuming!! And what this means is that you're very capable of being sexy, getting sexy, without the alcohol, plus are likelier to have a better time and one you can actually clearly remember!!

Your Brain on Booze

When alcohol and sex mix, the organ most affected is the brain. This happens because alcohol acts as a central nervous system depressant that, in turn, dulls the higher brain functions that normally control or inhibit sexual impulses. Alcohol loosens your inhibitions and impairs judgment. It is a depressant that can make you feel lonely and increase your desire for companionship and sexual contact.

Yet while alcohol may increase your desire to have sex, it *decreases* your ability to perform. Moderate to large quantities of alcohol rapidly lead to an inability to function sexually. Alcohol can cause problems with coordination, which can make having sex difficult. Plus, it inhibits clear thinking, makes talking and listening more difficult, and makes it harder to assess risk.

Many people have found that sex while drunk or buzzed just isn't all that. David says it flat-out:

> Drinking does nothing good for me sexually. I've never had good sex when drunk. It doesn't help at all. It makes sex more accessible, but the quality isn't as good. I don't think about sex any more or less when drunk. I'm a pretty reserved person and under normal circumstances, I wouldn't hit on somebody, but alcohol makes it more of a possibility. When I'm drunk, I always lose sensitivity. I can become a marathon man, but that doesn't make sex any more fun. It's not an aphrodisiac.

Women and Alcohol

Females actually have lower arousal levels when between the influence of alcohol and have greater difficulty achieving orgasm. It takes just one to two drinks for a woman's vaginal blood volume to begin to wane and for her orgasms to come more slowly. Over time, heavy alcohol use by a woman can lead to problems with her menstruation and sexual functioning. Lise knows the difficulty alcohol can have on a female's system: "Alcohol has major adverse affects on sexual functioning. It makes you want to do it more, but you are able to do it less."

In studies on sex and alcohol, women have reported that sexual pleasure increases as their blood alcohol level increases, despite the decreased blood volume that is being sent to the vagina that should really be lessening sexual feeling. Once again, that brain is simply amazing. Even as sexual activity declines with drinking, many women still report that drinking enhances their desire.

Liz, a 28-year-old nurse practitioner, believes that when drinking alcohol, sometimes it is a case of mind over matter: "Alcohol has always been an enhancer for me. I can be shy—even with people I know. Alcohol makes me far less inhibited socially and sexually. I am more of an aggressor when I am drinking, which pleases my partner. I also have a higher success of orgasm during intercourse when I am drinking."

Sarah, on the other hand, finds alcohol a bit of a handicap in the long run:

> I definitely become much less inhibited when I'm drinking. Many of my insecurities, especially body image, that normally make their way into the bedroom become less evident or nonexistent when I drink. I usually want sex more, but it's more about wanting to pleasure another person since my body tends to get numb, making it difficult for me to feel much or to have an orgasm. There's also a fine line for me. A little alcohol and I'm ready for sex. A lot and I am ready to sleep!

One survey found that as many as 30 percent of men and 14 percent of women have tried to get a person drunk or high in order to have sex with them.

Men and Alcohol

"Commander, we have a problem." For many men, sex while under the influence of alcohol is all about difficulty in achieving and maintaining an erection. After just two to three drinks, penile swelling begins to taper off. Demi recalls alcohol's negative effects on one of her past partners: "With my ex-boyfriend, we'd go out drinking and stuff and later, about 30 to 40 percent of the time, he could never get hard, especially if he'd smoked up too."

The higher his blood alcohol level, the longer it takes for a guy to ejaculate. For men at the highest levels of alcohol saturation, climax is almost impossible. In addition, heavy drinking over time can lead to health problems, like decreased sexual desire, increased estrogen levels (causing feminine characteristics in men, like loss of body hair and muscle mass), shrinking testicles, impotence, sperm deformities, decreased testosterone levels, and swollen breasts.

About three quarters of college students have had sex with someone who was drunk or high.

The Risks Involved with Drinking

One major concern about alcohol and sex is that people under the influence are at a higher risk for exercising bad judgment, which can lead to an increase in risk-taking behaviors. Johann exemplifies this pretty well in telling us about the time he lost his virginity:

> I totally regret my first time. We were both inebriated and I was clueless as to what I was doing—inexperienced. And she wasn't. I felt uncomfortable about that. I didn't know what I was doing and it was unprotected. I regret that. It wasn't that great. She wasn't very responsive and that didn't help me out as far as becoming a veteran sex machine.

With alcohol and sex stories like Johann's being common, it should come as no surprise to anybody that alcohol consumption is associated with unsafe sexual behaviors, and thus it increases your risk of contracting STDs and HIV. Likewise, sexual encounters with new partners are more likely to involve alcohol.

Having attended a large party school, Lacie mulls over just how risky her old sorority drinking days were:

> Drinking definitely allows you to be more experimental and feel more comfortable with your performance if you are a female. I know that I had a lot easier time hooking up when I was in college after I had drunk a little. I would never get to the point when drinking that I felt I had lost control of myself, though. I always had to know exactly what I was doing and with whom. A lot of crazy things went on at my undergraduate institution and I felt bad for the girls who got so drunk they would hook up with strangers and not remember what they did the next day.

Your risk of acquiring an STD while drunk and screwing around can double, due to the fact that even if you are using protection, it's likely that you'll be clumsier and more careless with the condoms, lube, and other devices.

For both men and women, heavier drinking patterns are associated with multiple sexual partners, being non-monogamous, or being with a non-monogamous partner. People who use illicit drugs or who have engaged in heavy drinking also tend to be those with a history of high rates of partner change and are also more likely than others to be in a risky sexual relationship.

Forty-one percent of men and 32 percent of women have had sex with someone they didn't like. Why? Most responded that it just happened, while the second most popular answer was that they were drunk or high.

Alcohol and Rape

Alcohol use by the victim or perpetrator is often associated with acquaintance rape. On average, 75 percent of male perpetrators and at least 55 percent of female victims are "mildly buzzed" to completely intoxicated or high at the time of a sexual assault.

Once again, beliefs and expectations play a role in these alcohol scenarios. After drinking alcohol, men expect to feel more powerful, sexual, and aggressive. Expectations like this can have a power of their own, independent of the alcohol's impact on the body. Research has shown that males who believe they have consumed alcohol, regardless of the actual drink content, show increased arousal to deviant stimuli, like rape and violent erotica.

So while the alcohol is affecting men in this manner, it is also doing a number on the women. In terms of effect, *consider that two drinks for a male is equivalent to one for a female.* So while she's trying to keep up with her male companion consumption-wise, a woman who is drinking may miss or ignore cues that suggest that an assault is likely, e.g., a guy is trying to get her to an isolated location or is encouraging her to drink even more so he can take advantage of her later. A woman who's been drinking may not realize that her friendly behavior is being perceived as seduction. Ultimately, alcohol consumption also decreases the female's likelihood of successfully verbally or physically resisting an assault.

To complicate this further, there are many stereotypes about women who drink alcohol. Among them is that women who drink alcohol are more sexually available than women who don't drink, that they are more willing to be seduced, and that they are more likely to engage in sexual intercourse. People view women who drink as being significantly more aggressive, sexually available, physically and mentally impaired, less attractive, and more likely to engage in sex play. Views like this really piss me off, but they're there and influence many sexual scenarios that involve alcohol.

> Studies have shown that 40 percent of men feel that it is acceptable to force sex on a drunk date. In a study on acknowledged date rapists, 75 percent admitted that they sometimes got women drunk in order to increase the likelihood of having sex with them.

With such a high number of men admitting to this, it's ironic that women who are drunk when raped are often viewed by others as at least partially responsible for what happened. Since she is responsible for her drinking, and drinking shows bad judgment, people often hold the female victim responsible for the rape incident, as was the case with Arien:

> When I was sexually assaulted, I was so inebriated that I can hardly remember the incident at all. It took me a while to want to see it as rape. One of the reasons for this was that when I told my buddy Will that this guy had had sex with me when I was absolutely hammered, and I didn't know what to make of it since I couldn't remember much, other than that I was crying hysterically, his reaction was, "Arien, why do you always seem to let things like this happen to you?!" Immediately, I disregarded the thought that it was rape since I must've been at fault for "allowing" myself to get so drunk that a guy could take advantage of me.

Furthermore, alcohol consumption by men is likely to enhance the chance that misperception will occur and lead to sexual assault. When intoxicated, it is easy for a man to ignore a woman's reluctance and her "No's," and to force sex on an unwilling partner. This is especially likely when a man feels justified in forcing sex on a woman who, he believes, has been leading him on or who is a sexual tease.

> Studies show that men are more likely than women to interpret a variety of verbal and nonverbal cues as evidence that a female is interested in having sex. For example, studies have shown that men are more likely than women to rate revealing clothing; drinking alcohol; complimenting a date; secluded date locations, like the beach or his room; and tickling a date as indicative of a desire to have sexual intercourse.

WHAT IS GOING TOO FAR?

＊ If you're too drunk to understand a person trying to say "No."

* If you're too drunk to listen and respect a person trying to say "No."

* If you have sex with a person who is incapable of giving consent.

When you drink you need to be in control of yourself, responsible for your behavior, even if you're trashed. Byron says it well:

> Beer goggles—don't know if they exist. Maybe they do. Alcohol can affect your ability to become erect or control ejaculation—that's for sure. It lowers your inhibitions. For me, with alcohol, it's important to remember that it lowers inhibitions. A guy can be raw, a Neanderthal man, and want to have sex. Guys need to remember that the rules of the game still apply, even if you've had a drink—that you should still treat her like a lady.

Drinking is *not* an excuse for misbehaving or forcing sex upon a person. Although alcohol may help you rationalize sex and sexually aggressive behaviors, drunk or sober, rape is rape. Giving consent means having the ability to make a decision. Having sex with a person who is mentally or physically incapable of giving consent is rape. If a person has passed out, or isn't in control of herself/himself, having sex with that person is rape.

Date-Rape Drugs

Date-rape drugs are becoming more and more common at bar and club scenes and are being used more and more often by rapists. I want to touch on the two predominant date-rape drugs so you know what you need to be wary of when you're living it up.

ROHYPNOL: THE "DATE-RAPE DRUG"

Rohypnol is often referred to as the "date-rape drug" because men at bars, clubs, and social events drop it into women's drinks where it quickly dissolves, and eventually causes the drinker to black out. This illegal drug creates the perfect opportunity for a rape situation, especially since the woman will have no recollection of the events that occur while she's under the influence of Rohypnol. Thus, the woman can't remember what happened, may feel a little sluggish and think that she drank too much the night before, and have difficulty remembering anything, since her night was a series of blackouts.

Only ten minutes after ingesting Rohypnol, a person may begin to feel dizzy, disoriented, too hot and too cold, and nauseated. She may then have difficulty speaking, followed by passing out. Sedation occurs twenty to thirty minutes after administration of a 2mg pill and lasts for about eight to twelve hours. When mixed with alcohol or other drugs, Rohypnol can cause respiratory depression, coma, and death.

> It was a mixture of Rohypnol and champagne that sent rock star Kurt Cobain of Nirvana into a coma one month before he committed suicide.

GHB—GAMMA-HYDROXYBUTYRATE

GHB ("liquid X," "g-juice") is another colorless, odorless, date-rape drug that is being used to incapacitate victims in order to sexually assault them. GHB, which is most commonly found in liquid form, was once sold in health food stores to bodybuilders since it was thought to help stimulate muscle growth. As soon as its bad side effects—like dizziness, confusion, and memory loss—were realized, it was pulled off the market. This dangerous, illegal drug is inexpensive and easy to obtain, making it a frighteningly powerful weapon in the hands of a potential rapist.

TIPS TO HELP YOU REDUCE YOUR RISK OF ALCOHOL-RELATED SEXUAL ASSAULT

* Do not leave your beverages unattended at a bar or party.

* Do not take any kind of beverage from someone you do not know well or trust.

* Limit your alcohol consumption.

* Try not to mix different types of alcoholic beverages at one time. Mixing may accelerate sedating effects.

* Make arrangements with a friend so that you leave together when drinking in social settings.

* Drink on a full stomach to help reduce sedating effects.

* Drink soda, water, or juice after an alcoholic drink.

* Eat food while you're drinking.

Determine how much alcohol you can handle and still be in control of yourself, keeping in mind that the number of drinks consumed per hour is significant. Remember that the concentration of alcohol in your blood depends on the following:

* the amount of alcohol you're consuming (and its strength)

* the length of time that you've been drinking

* the presence/absence of food in your stomach

* your metabolism

Drinking in moderation can be a nice thing to do. It may even be beneficial in that it may decrease some people's inhibitions and thus increase their sexual desire. Men with very low blood alcohol levels (.025 percent) actually achieve maximum penile diameter. So if you're going to drink, try to limit yourself to two drinks. Just four ounces of alcohol can make a man lose his erection and cause a woman to have difficulty attaining orgasm, plus can cause people to incorrectly use birth control and condoms.

I know that I came across in this chapter as rather anti-alcohol. But I want you to know what really goes on with your body and social circle when you drink, and I want you to look out for your health, equipped with facts versus fallacies. So cheers to you and to that!

RESOURCES

For more information on rape and sexual assault, call or visit the following:

Center for Disease Control Rape Hotline: (800) 656-4673

Rape, Abuse, Incest National Network (RAINN): (800) 656-HOPE (656-4673) or www.RAINN.org

CHAPTER 19

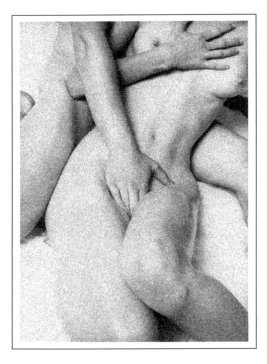

In Conclusion

I hope that you had as good a time reading this book as I had writing it. It was my pet for a year, taking priority over most things in my life, and I think that it was a year well spent. I'm a big advocate for access to information; all of you have a right to know everything we've just covered. You have a right not only to look out for your sexual health, but also to eroticize your sexuality. Don't let anyone ever tell you otherwise!

Right after finishing this book, I was in a Boston metro station with my friend Jon. A couple of older men, carrying religious billboards, were preaching to the crowd about the sins of premarital sex. On hearing that I'm a sex educator, one of them got in my face and screamed, "Damn you, sinnerrrrr!!! You're going to helllll! Repent while you cannnnn!!" Jon and I just laughed, but really, what a price I'm going to pay for writing this book! I think it'll be worth it, though. I hope you think so too.

As a sex educator, I have to have a sense of humor about such incidents. Sometimes it's the only way to deal with people who don't respect others' sexual beliefs, decisions, practices, and desires. Sometimes it's the only way to deal with people who don't want you to know the entire array of all of your sexuality-related choices. While we don't have to agree with what other people do between the sheets, we should respect it. Don't ever be afraid to make that clear to others.

I leave you with a parable about a couple of boys who want to play a practical joke on an old lady. One kid has a bird in his hands and he says to the other, "Let's go ask the old lady if the bird in my hands is alive or dead. If she says it's dead, I'll open my hands and let it fly free, but if she says that it's alive, then I'll crush it to death!"

So the two approach the old lady and the boy poses his question, "Tell me, old lady, is the bird in my hands dead or alive?" The old lady stares at him long and hard. She stares at him and stares at him and stares at him and stares at him some more, and finally says, "The answer...is in your hands."

The answers to all of your sexual-health decisions are in your hands. You decide your fate. You decide if you're going to have safer sex, solo sex, or no sex. You decide if you're going to protect yourself. You decide if you're going to eroticize your sex play. You deal the deck of cards and play your hand.

Glossary

Abstinence—in sexual terms, refraining from all sexual activity that involves the exchange of bodily fluids, e.g., penile–vaginal intercourse

Acquired immune deficiency syndrome (AIDS)—a disease, caused by HIV, which destroys the body's natural immunity and increases its susceptibility to unusual forms of cancer and infection

Acyclovir—a drug used to treat herpes infections

Afterplay—post-sex touch and play

AIDS—*See* Acquired immune deficiency syndrome

AIDS-related complex (ARC)—a condition in which signs or symptoms of HIV infection appear, yet the individual falls short of having a full-blown AIDS case

Amenorrhea—a lack of menstruation

Anal beads—plastic or latex beads strung together on a nylon or cotton cord that are used for anal sex play

Anal intercourse—a sexual behavior involving insertion of one person's penis into another's anus

Analingus—stimulation of the anus with the mouth

Anterior Fornix Erogenous Zone—*See* A-spot

Anus—the rectal opening located between the buttocks

Aphrodisiac—a food, drink, drug, scent, or device that is believed to arouse or increase one's sexual desire, libido, and attraction

ARC—*See* AIDS-related complex

Areola—the dark, circular skin that surrounds the nipple of the breast

Arousal Stage—first stage of the sexual response cycle, a.k.a. the "Excitement Phase"

A-spot—smooth area midway between the woman's cervix and G-spot, on the anterior wall of the vagina, that appears as a spongy, wrinkled, scrotal-like swelling and that is extremely sensitive to stimulating touch, a.k.a. "Anterior Fornix Erogenous Zone"

Asymptomatic—without symptoms

Autoeroticism—self-stimulation, e.g., masturbation

Bacterial Vaginosis (BV)—a vaginal bacterial infection, caused by an overgrowth of various bacteria, that is marked by a malodorous grayish-white discharge, burning, and itching

Barrier methods—contraceptives designed to block sperm from entering the uterus, e.g., cervical cap

Bartholin's glands—two small glands, just inside the inner lips of the vagina, that secrete a small amount of fluid during sexual stimulation, a.k.a. "Greater Vestibular Glands"

Basal Body Temperature (BBT)—natural family planning method involving a woman taking her temperature immediately after awakening to predict her ovulation

Ben wa balls—small, solid metal balls inserted into the vagina for sexual stimulation

Birth control—devices or techniques used to prevent the union of sperm and eggs in order to avoid pregnancy

Birth control pills—a.k.a. "the pill"; hormones a woman takes daily to prevent ovulation and, hence, pregnancy

Bisexual—a person sexually attracted to both males and females

Body image—a person's self-image, attitudes, and feelings about his or her body and appearance

Breasts—In females, the secondary sex organs found on the chest, composed of fatty and fibrous tissue, that surround fifteen to twenty clusters of mammary glands. In males, another term for chest.

Bulbourethral glands—two pea-sized glands on either side of the male's urethra, a.k.a. "Cowper's glands," that secrete pre-ejaculatory fluid

Butt plug—a dildo specially designed for anal and rectal pleasure via insertion into the anus

Calendar method—a form of the rhythm method during which a woman monitors the days of her menstrual cycle to determine when the risk of pregnancy is low

Candidiasis—a fungal or yeast infection of the genitals or rectum

Cervical cap—a thimble-shaped, small plastic or rubber contraceptive device that is inserted into the vagina before sex and that fits snugly over the cervix to prevent sperm from entering the uterus

Cervical mucus method—a natural family planning method of birth control that involves monitoring vaginal mucus changes to determine a woman's most (or least) fertile periods

Cervical Os—a very small opening to the cervix; the point where menstrual flow exits the uterus and sperm cells enter it

Cervix—opening to the lower part of uterus that protrudes into the vagina

Chancre—a painless sore, which is an early sign of syphilis, with a hard ridge around it

Chancroid—an ulcer on or about the genitals, caused by a bacteria that is sexually transmitted

Chlamydia—a bacterial sexually transmitted infection; symptoms include painful urination and/or genital discharge

Climax—orgasm

Clitoral hood—a sheath of tissue that protects the clitoris and is an extension of the inner lips that run alongside the vaginal opening

Clitoris—the female's highly sensitive sexual organ, located in front of the vaginal entrance and urethra, that is filled with a high number of nerve endings

Cock ring—a rubber, metal, or leather band worn around the base of the penis for sex play

Coitus—insertion of the penis into the vagina; sexual intercourse

Coitus interruptus—*See* Withdrawal method

Combination pill—a birth control pill containing both estrogen and progesterone

Condom—a latex, polyurethane, or sheepskin disposable sheath placed over an erect penis, which acts as a barrier to prevent pregnancy and the spread of STDs and HIV

Corona—a raised ridge separating the glans from the body of penis; the most sexually excitable region of penis

Cowper's clands—*See* Bulbourethral glands

Crabs—*See* Pediculosis pubis

Cunnilingus—stimulation of the female genitals with the mouth

Dental dam—latex or Saran Wrap barrier placed over the vagina or anus during sexual activity to prevent the spread of STDs

Depo-Provera—used as a form of birth control in women; a drug containing the hormone progestin, administered in shots every three months

Detumescence—loss of the male erection

Diaphragm—a dome-shaped, rubber contraceptive device that fits inside a woman's vagina, over the cervix, and that blocks the sperm from entering the uterus

Dildo—a sex toy, made of rubber, silicone, or latex, that can be inserted into the vagina or anus

Egg—the female reproductive cell

Ejaculation—the sudden, forceful discharge of semen out of the penis

Ejaculatory inevitability—the sensation that ejaculation is about to happen and cannot be stopped; the "point of no return" or the end of the "control zone"

Emergency contraceptive pill (ECP)—an intense dose of progestin-only birth control pills or combined pills, taken seventy-two hours after unprotected sex, that can prevent a pregnancy

Endometrium—inner layer of the uterus, which thickens with blood and then sloughs off when a woman has her menstrual period, or in which the fertilized egg implants

Epididymis—a tightly coiled, thin tube that lies alongside and on top of testicles where sperm spend several weeks maturing

Erection—an enlargement of the penis that occurs when blood flows to the area

Erogenous zones—areas of the body that are particularly sensitive to sexual stimulation

Excitement phase—the first phase of the sexual response cycle, characterized by increasing levels of myotonia and vasocongestion

Fallopian tube—a tube extending from the uterus to the ovary that transports the eggs from the ovaries to the uterus

Fellatio—stimulation of the male genitals with the mouth

Female condom—a disposable, polyurethane contraceptive tube, with a plastic ring at each end, that is inserted into the vagina to prevent pregnancy and the transmission of STDs and HIV

Female ejaculation—the phenomenon of prostatic-like fluid being expelled during G-spot stimulation and/or orgasm

Fertility awareness methods (FAM)—natural methods of birth control involving the prediction of a woman's fertile period, based on changes in her body temperature and cervical mucus

Flaccid—not erect

Foreplay—sexual stimulation that takes place before intercourse

Foreskin—in uncircumcised males, the layer of skin covering the glans that retracts when the male is aroused and erect

Frenulum—a tiny band of skin near the indentation on the underside of penis where the glans meets the shaft

Gamma-Hydroxybutyrate (GHB)—colorless, odorless "date-rape drug"

Gay—term referring to a male who is sexually attracted to other males or a female who is attracted to females; synonymous with "homosexual"

Genital Warts—*See* Human Papilloma Virus

Genitals—the sexual or reproductive organs

Glans—in the male, the smooth, extremely sensitive tip (head) of the penis that contains numerous nerve endings; in the female, the extremely sensitive, visible external tip of the clitoris that protrudes like a small lump

Gluteal sex—sexual activity involving the man thrusting the crease of his partner's buttocks

Gonad—ovary or testicle

Gonorrhea—a bacterial sexually transmitted infection with symptoms that include vaginal discharge, burning urination, fever, and pelvic-area pain

Gräfenberg Spot—*See* G-spot

Groin—the area where the thigh joins the abdomen

G-spot—a small mass of erectile nerve tissue, ducts, glands, and blood vessels located between pubic bone and front of cervix

Hepatitis—a viral sexually transmitted infection, with several different strains, causing liver damage, that can be transmitted via anal intercourse or analingus

Herpes—a viral sexually transmitted infection with two strains: herpes simplex type-1 (oral herpes) and herpes simplex type-2 (genital herpes), both of which cause blisters or sores on the given area

Heterosexual—a person who is sexually attracted to members of the other gender

HIV—*See* Human immunodeficiency virus

Homosexual—a person who is sexually attracted to members of his or her own gender

Hormones—chemicals produced by certain glands in the body

Human immunodeficiency virus (HIV)—the retrovirus that causes AIDS

Human papilloma virus (HPV)—a viral sexually transmitted infection that can produce warts on the genitals, a.k.a. "genital warts"

Hymen—a thin tissue membrane that covers the opening of vagina on some women

Inner Lips—*See* Labia minora

Intercourse—*See* Sexual intercourse

Interfemoral sex—sexual activity involving the man thrusting between his partner's thighs

Intrauterine device (IUD)—a small, plastic or metal contraceptive device that is inserted into the uterus to prevent pregnancy

Kegel exercises—contractions performed to strengthen the PC muscle surrounding the genitals

Labia majora—rounded pads of fatty and fibrous tissue, covered with pubic hair, that lie on either side of the vaginal entrance

Labia minora—thin folds of skin that lie on either side of the vaginal entrance and extend forward to come together in front of the clitoris to form the clitoral hood

Latent phase—third stage in the course of syphilis, when symptoms disappear and the disease is no longer contagious

Lesbian—a woman who is sexually attracted to other women

Libido—sex drive

Lunelle—a shot of combined hormones administered in a female's arm, buttocks, or thigh every month for contraception

Masturbation—self-stimulation of the genitals with the hand or an object

Ménage à trois—sexual activity involving three people

Menstruation—monthly bloody discharge of the uterine lining

Million-dollar point—indentation on male's perineum, just in front of his anus, that, when pushed, can help to stop ejaculation

Minipill—birth control pill containing a low dose of progesterone and no estrogen

Monogamy—the state of being sexual with only one person over a period of time

Mons pubis—the fatty pad of tissue and skin under a woman's pubic hair, over her pubic bone, which is thought to protect her pubic bones from damage during vigorous sexual thrusting

"Morning-after pill"—*See* Emergency contraceptive pill

Mucous membranes—the soft, wet linings of the mouth, nose, eyes, anus, and vagina

Multiple orgasms—a series of orgasmic responses that occur without dropping below the plateau level of arousal

Myometrium—the muscular, middle layer of uterus that provides it with strength during childbirth

Myotonia—a muscle contraction

Natural family planning—methods of birth control that involve abstaining from sexual intercourse during the fertile days of a woman's menstrual cycle

Nipple—the pigmented tip of the breast, through which milk passes when a woman is breast-feeding, containing erectile tissue that may provide sexual pleasure when stimulated

Nocturnal orgasm—involuntary orgasm, most often accompanied with emission in males, that occurs during sleep

Nongonococcal urethritis (NGU)—inflammation of the male's urethra not caused by gonorrhea

Norplant—an implanted, progestin-only contraceptive for females

NuvaRing—small, flexible ring inserted deep into vagina for three weeks each month that releases combined hormones that protect against pregnancy

Oral contraceptives—birth control pills, containing the hormone progestin and/or estrogen, that prevent a woman from ovulating

Oral sex—sexual activity involving mouth stimulation of the genitals

Orgasm—a series of involuntary muscular contractions and a feeling of intense pleasure focused in the genitals that peak at sexual arousal and that may spread throughout the body; third and shortest phase of the sexual response cycle

Orgasmic platform—during sexual arousal, a thickening of the walls of the outer third of the vagina

Orthro-Evra—see Patch

Outer lips—*See* Labia majora

Ovaries—found at either end of the fallopian tubes, two organs that produce eggs that are released at ovulation and the sex hormones estrogen and progesterone

Ovulation—release of an egg by the ovaries

Pap test—the test for cervical cancer during a gynecological exam in which cells are taken from the cervix and vagina and examined under a microscope

Patch—a thin, plastic patch placed on skin of a woman's buttocks, stomach, upper outer arm, or upper torso, once per week for three weeks each month. The patch releases combined hormones to protect against pregnancy

PC muscle—*See* Pubococcygeus muscle

Pediculosis pubis—a parasitic sexually transmitted infection of lice attaching themselves to the roots of the pubic hairs; "crabs"

Pelvic inflammatory disease (PID)—an infection of the pelvic organs

Penis—the male reproductive and sex organ which passes sperm into the vagina and urine out of the body

Perineum—a soft, hairless tissue between the genitals and anus in both sexes

Periodic abstinence—temporarily refraining from sex at times

Plateau phase—the second phase of the sexual response cycle, just before orgasm

Polyurethane condom—a plastic barrier, worn over an erect penis, that prevents pregnancy and the spread of STDs

Pornography—erotic materials meant to sexually arouse

Pre-cum—*See* Pre-ejaculatory fluid

Pre-ejaculatory fluid—a clear, alkaline fluid, secreted by the Cowper's glands, that appears at the tip of the penis before a man ejaculates

Prostate—gland found under the bladder and behind the pubic bone, just under the perineum, that secretes some of the milky, alkaline fluid in semen

Prostatitis—a prostate gland inflammation due to infection

Pubic Lice—*See* Pediculosis pubis

Pubococcygeus muscle (PC muscle)—the muscle that extends from the pubic bone, around both sides of the sex organ, and back to the tailbone

Pudendum—another term for "vulva"

Rape—oral, vaginal, or anal penetration that is nonconsensual and obtained by force, threat of bodily harm, or when the victim is incapable of giving consent

Rape trauma syndrome—collection of emotional and physical effects a victim experiences following a rape or an attempted rape

Rectum—lower part of the large intestine

Refractory period—period following male orgasm during which he cannot be sexually aroused

Resolution phase—the final stage of the sexual response cycle, which occurs after orgasm, when the body returns to its unaroused, pre-excitement state

Rhythm method—a birth control method that involves abstaining from sexual intercourse during the fertile days of a female's menstrual cycle

Rimming—*See* Analingus

Rohypnol—a "date-rape drug"; used to sedate a person without her knowledge, and commonly used prior to a sexual assault on the person

Root—part of the penis that attaches to the body

RU-486—a pill that produces an early abortion

Safer sex—vaginal, anal, or oral sex involving practices that reduce the risk of pregnancy, HIV, and STDs

Scabies—a contagious skin disease spread through sexual contact or contaminated sheets or towels

Scrotum—the pouch of skin, containing numerous sebaceous glands and hair, that holds the testicles

Semen—fluid, containing sperm, that is ejaculated from the penis

Seminal vesicles—two small sacs that produce and secrete about 60 percent of semen

Seminiferous tubules—tiny, coiled tubes in the testes that produce sperm

Sex toy—an object used to enhance sexual activity

Sexual dysfunction—condition in which the ordinary physical responses of sexual excitement and orgasm are impaired, whether because of psychosocial or physical reasons

Sexual identity—how a person thinks of him/herself in terms of his/her sexual orientation, based upon whom he or she is sexually and romantically attracted to

Sexual intercourse—sexual activity in which the penis is inserted into the vagina; for some, is defined as sexual activity in which the penis is inserted into the anus, or fingers or a sex toy are inserted into the vagina or anus

Sexual orientation—who a person is sexually and romantically attracted to; usually designated as "heterosexual," "bisexual," or "homosexual" ("straight," "bi," or "gay")

Sexual response cycle—the stages an individual experiences physically and psychologically when engaging in sexual activity

Sexually transmitted disease (STD)—any disease that can be transmitted via sexual contact

Sexually transmitted infection (STI)—*See* Sexually transmitted disease

Shaft—in the male, the part of the penis that runs between the glans and root; in the female, the part of the clitoris that disappears into the body beneath the clitoral hood

Sheepskin condom—a barrier, made of lamb intestines, worn over an erect penis that helps to prevent pregnancy and the spread of STDs

Simultaneous orgasm—when both partners experience orgasm at the same time

Sixty-nine—sexual position that allows oral stimulation of the genitals of both partners at the same time

Skene's glands—the female's urethral glands that secrete female ejaculatory fluid in women who ejaculate

Soixante-neuf—French for "sixty-nine"; *See* Sixty-nine

Sperm—the mature male reproductive cell, capable of fertilizing an egg

Spermicide—a substance that kills sperm

Sponge—a polyurethane-foam birth control device that fits over the cervix

Spontaneous orgasm—orgasm without any genital contact, a.k.a. "Extragenital Orgasm"

Syphilis—a bacterial sexually transmitted infection, with three stages of symptoms

Temperature method—birth control technique to determine the part of the menstrual cycle during which pregnancy is likely to occur so that intercourse can then be avoided

Tertiary phase—*See* Latent phase

Testes—the male gonads; a pair of oval glands in the scrotum, which manufacture sperm and sex hormones, primarily testosterone, a.k.a. "testicles"

Testicle—a testis

Threesome—*See* Ménage à trois

Toxic shock syndrome (TSS)—a rare disease, which can be fatal, associated with prolonged tampon use or with prolonged use of some barrier methods of contraception

Trichomoniasis—a vaginal infection

Urethra—a slender tube acting as a passageway for urine or semen making its way out of the body; in a woman, it runs parallel to the vagina

Urethral opening—an acorn-shaped protrusion found between the clitoris and vaginal opening

Urethral sponge—spongy, erectile tissue, which contains the paraurethral glans and ducts, a.k.a. "G-spot"

Urinary tract infection (UTI)—an infection of the urinary tract that causes burning during urination and an urgency to urinate

Uterus—the hollow, muscular organ located in abdomen, a.k.a. "womb," where a fetus develops

Vagina—highly muscular, three- to four-inch long, tube-shaped organ in the female that is penetrated during sex, and through which a baby passes during birth

Vaginal cone—a weighted device, inserted into the vagina, used during pelvic-floor muscle exercises

Vaginal opening—the entrance, leading from the outside into the female's vagina, through which a baby passes during birth and through which menstrual blood passes during a woman's period

Vas deferens—tubes that transport sperm to seminal vesicles and the prostate gland from the epididymis

Vasocongestion—the accumulation of blood in the blood vessels of a region of the body, especially the genitals and breasts

Venereal disease—old term for "sexually transmitted infection"

Viagra—pill used to treat male erectile dysfunction

Vibrator—a battery-operated or electric device that vibrates to stimulate body parts, particularly the genitals

Virgin—a person who has never had sex, whether that is personally defined as oral, anal, or vaginal–penile intercourse

Vulva—a collective term for the female external genitals: the clitoris, mons pubis, labia minora, labia majora, urethral opening, and vaginal opening

Wet dream—*see* Nocturnal orgasm

Withdrawal method—a practice, sometimes used as a birth control method, during which a male withdraws his penis from the vagina before he ejaculates

Yeast infection—a vaginal bacterial infection involving a cottage cheese–like discharge

Resources

Books

Bodansky, Steve, and Vera Bodansky. *Extended Massive Orgasm: How You Can Give and Receive Intense Sexual Pleasure*. Alameda, CA: Hunter House, 2000.

Bodansky, Steve, and Vera Bodansky. *The Illustrated Guide to Extended Massive Orgasm*. Alameda, CA: Hunter House, 2002.

Chia, Mantak, and Douglas Abrams. *The Multi-Orgasmic Man.* San Francisco, CA: HarperCollins, 1996.

Craze, Richard. *The Pocket Book of Sex and Chocolate*. Alameda, CA: Hunter House, 2001.

Dodson, Betty. *Sex for One: The Joy of Selfloving*. Westminster, MD: Harmony Books, 1986. Reissued New York: Three Rivers Press, 1996.

Federation of Feminist Women's Health Care Centers, *A New View of a Woman's Body*, Second Edition. Illustrated by Suzan Gage. Los Angeles, CA: Feminist Health Press, 1991.

Keesling, Barbara, Ph.D. *Rx Sex: Making Love Is the Best Medicine*. Alameda, CA: Hunter House, 2000.

Keesling, Barbara, Ph.D. *Sexual Healing: A Self-Help Program to Enhance Your Sensuality and Overcome Common Sexual Problems*. Alameda, CA: Hunter House, 1990.

Keesling, Barbara, Ph.D. *Sexual Pleasure: Reaching New Heights of Sexual Arousal and Intimacy*. Alameda, CA: Hunter House, 1993.

Organizations and Websites

CHAPTER 4: You Always Can in Fantasyland

Gay and Lesbian National Hotline: (888) THE-GLNH
Website: www.glnh.org
If you're wondering whether you're gay, straight, or bisexual, or if you've determined that you're gay or lesbian and are looking for support in coming to terms with that realization or breaking the news to others, contact this organization.

Gay Men's Health Crisis Hotline: (800) AIDS NYC (243-7692)

CHAPTER 6: Who Me? Get an STD?

ASHA—American Social Health Association
PO Box 13827
Research Triangle Park NC 27709
(919) 361-8400   Fax: (919) 361-8425
Website: www.ashastd.org
A nonprofit organization offering STD information

Centers for Disease Control
National STD Hotline: (800) 227-8922
Website: http://www.cdc.gov/netinfo.htm

Herpes Advice Center: (888) ADVICE8 (238-4238)

Herpes Information Resource: www.herpes.com

The Herpes Zone: www.herpeszone.com

Herpes & HPV Hotline: (800) 230-6039

HPV Hotline: (877) HPV-5868 (478-5868) (toll free), 2:00–7:00 P.M. EST

www.thebody.com: For information on STDs

http://thebody.com/sowadsky/symptoms/symptoms.html: To learn to identify STDs by sight

CHAPTER 7: The Lowdown on HIV/AIDS

American Social Health Association
PO Box 13827
Research Triangle Park NC 27709
(919) 361-8400   Fax: (919) 361-8425
Website: www.ashastd.org

National AIDS Hotline: (800) 342-AIDS (342-2437) or www.ashastd.org

HIV/AIDS Treatment Information Service: (800) 448-0440

AZT Hotline at the National Institutes of Health: (800) 843-9388

Centers for Disease Control and Prevention National Prevention Information Network: www.cdcnpin.org

 Public Health Service Hotline: (800) 342-AIDS (342-2437)

AIDS Education Global Information System: www.aegis.com

CHAPTER 8: Gettin' Jiggy with Contraception: The Bare Essentials of Pregnancy and STD Prevention

Birth Control information: www.birthcontrol.com

Condom information: www.condoms.net/?TO=/condoms/how_to_use.html

Condomania: www.condomania.com

Contraception information: (888) PREVEN2 (773-8362)

Emergency Contraception Hotline: (888) Not-2-LATE (668-2528)

National Abortion Federation Hotline: (800) 772-9100

National Adoption Clearinghouse: (301) 231-6512

National Pregnancy Hotline: (800) 311-2229

NARAL on state abortion laws: www.naral.org

Planned Parenthood Federation of America
434 West 33rd St.
New York NY 10001   (800) 230-PLAN (230-7526)
(212) 541-7800   Fax: (212) 245-1845
Website: www.plannedparenthood.org or www.ppfa.org

CHAPTER 9: Something to Get Sexcited About: Safer Sex

American Social Health Association
PO Box 13827
Research Triangle Park NC 27709
(919) 361-8400   Fax: (919) 361-8425
Website: www.ashastd.org

National AIDS Hotline: (800) 342-AIDS (342-2437) or www.ashastd.org

Centers for Disease Control: www.cdc.gov or (800) 342-AIDS (342-2437)

Coalition for Positive Sexuality: www.positive.org

Planned Parenthood Federation of America
434 West 33rd St.
New York NY 10001   (800) 230-PLAN (230-7526)
(212) 541-7800   Fax: (212) 245-1845
Website: www.plannedparenthood.org or www.ppfa.org

The Rubber Tree: www.rubbertree.org
Nonprofit organization that sells interesting, safe, FDA-approved condoms.

The Society for Human Sexuality: Their "Comprehensive Guide to Safer Sex"
can be found on their website at www.sexuality.org

CHAPTER 14: You Want Something to Play With?

Eve's Garden
119 W. 57th St.
New York NY 10019   (800) 848-3837
Website: www.evesgarden.com

Good Vibrations
1210 Valencia St.
San Francisco CA 94110   (800) 289-8423
Website: www.goodvibes.com

Good Vibrations
1620 Polk St.
San Francisco CA 94109   (415) 345-0400

Good Vibrations
2504 San Pablo Blvd.
Berkeley CA 94702   (800) 289-8423

Grand Opening!
318 Harvard St., #32 Arcade Bldg.
Boston MA 02446   (877) 731-2626
Website: www.grandopening.com

Grand Opening!
8442 Santa Monica Blvd.
West Hollywood CA 90069   (323) 848-6970
mail order: (877) 731-2626

The Love Boutique
18637 Ventura Blvd.
Tarzana CA 91356   (818) 342-2400
Website: www.pleasurefaire.com

The Love Boutique
2924 Wilshire Blvd.
Santa Monica CA 90403   (310) 453-3459

Toys in Babeland
707 E. Pike St.
Seattle WA 98122   (800) 658-9119
Website: www.babeland.com

Toys in Babeland
94 Rivington St.
New York NY 10002   (800) 658-9119

Come As You Are
701 Queen's St. W.
Toronto Ontario, Canada   (877) 858-3160
Website: www.comeasyouare.com

Good For Her
175 Harbord St.
Toronto Ontario, Canada   (877) 588-0900
Website: www.goodforher.com

Adam and Eve catalog: (800) 274-0333 or www.adameve.com

Liberator Shapes: www.liberatorshapes.com

www.loveandintimacy.com

www.lovenectar.com

www.pleasurespot.com.au

www.secretgardenpublishing.com

www.tantra.com   (800) 982-6872

www.xandria.com

CHAPTER 17: Horny and High: What Drugs Really Do to Your Sex Life

Dance Safe Organization: www.dancesafe.org

Drug Abuse Hotline: (800) 821-4357

National Institute on Drug Abuse: www.nida.nih.gov

CHAPTER 18: Why Don't We Get Drunk and Screw?

Center for Disease Control Rape Hotline: (800) 656-4673

Rape, Abuse, Incest National Network (RAINN): (800) 656-HOPE (656-4673) or www.RAINN.org

Information about Yvonne K. Fulbright

To learn more about Yvonne as well as her projects, lectures, and media appearances, visit www.yvonnekfulbright.com

Index

Cowper's glands, 21f, 22, 307

crabs, 109–110, 313. See also STDs

crack, 288–289. See also drug use and sex

crystal meth, 289–290. See also drug use and sex

cunnilingus, 212–215, 309. See also oral sex

D

Dangerous Tides, 195. See also pornography

date-rape drugs, 301–303

Debbie Does Dallas: The Next Generation, 195. See also pornography

Depo-Provera, 158–160, 179–180f, 309. See also contraceptives

depression, contraceptive use and, 153, 159, 162, 166; following ecstasy use, 287; sex and, 24

desire, as a sexual response cycle stage, 24–25

detumescence, 27, 309. See also erection

diaphragm, description, 146–148, 309; G-spot stimulation and, 229; Kegel exercises and, 261. See also contraceptives

dildos, 253–254f, 309. See also toys; vibrators

dirty talk, description, 238–239; fantasies and, 243; how to do, 239–242, 240t, 241t; other noise in sex, 243–245; on the telephone, 245–246

discharge, chlamydia, 97t; gonorrhea, 94t; herpes, 103t; pelvic inflammatory disease, 101; vaginosis, 98–99t

doggie-style, 205f–206, 229. See also positions

domination, 62, 202–203

drug use and sex, cocaine, 288–289; crystal meth, 289–290; date-rape drugs, 301–303; description, 283, 291; ecstasy, 285–287; heroin, 290–291; marijuana, 284–285; poppers, 287–288. See also alcohol use and sex

E

"eating her out," 212–215. See also oral sex

ecstasy use and sex, 285–287. See also drug use and sex

ejaculation, condom use and, 137; control zone period, 268–269; controlling, 271–280; description, 309; female, 16, 230–231, 310; heroin use and, 290; history of, 48; HIV transmission and, 119–121; inevitability of, 26, 309; Kegel exercises and, 261–262; male, 21; orgasm and, 32; post-poning, 270–271; swallowing, 217–218; withdrawal method use and, 170–171. See also multi-orgasmic men; orgasm; pre-ejaculatory fluid

ejaculatory inevitability, 26, 309. See also ejaculation; orgasm

emergency contraception pills, 172–174, 309. See also contraceptives

emission phase of orgasm, 26, 270. See also orgasm

epididymis, 22, 309

erection, alcohol use and, 297, 303; cock rings and, 252–253f; condom use and, 138; description, 309; drug use and, 286, 288–289, 290; during a hand job, 219; Kegel exercises and, 262; multiple orgasms and, 41–42; during resolution stage, 27

erogenous zones, A-spot, 233–234; description, 235–236, 309. See also G-spot

erotic talk. See dirty talk

excitement stage, 25, 306, 309. See also sexual response cycle

expectations, 39–40, 294–295

expulsion stage of orgasm, 26–27, 270

extragenital orgasm, 35–36, 315. See also orgasm

eye contact, 72–73, 184

F

faking it, 43–45. See also orgasm

fallopian tube, 17f, 18, 309

fantasies, about the same sex, 63–64;

169–170, 178; description, 117–118, 311; drug use and, 283, 288, 289–290; mutual masturbation and, 219; oral sex and, 212, 218; protecting yourself, 122–124; safer sex and, 23, 124, 176–177; symptoms, 125; testing, 125–127; transmission of, 119–121. See also AIDS; safer sex; STDs

home pregnancy tests, 171–172. See also pregnancy

homophobia, anal sex and, 208

homosexuality, 64–65, 311

HPV, 104–106, 105t. See also STDs

human immunodeficiency virus. See HIV

human papilloma virus, 104–106, 105t, 178, 311. See also STDs

humor during sex, vaginal farts and, 203; while developing ejaculatory control, 278

hymen, 16–17, 311

I

ice, using during oral sex, 215

illness, sex and, 24

immune system, AIDS and, 119

Implanon, 164–165. See also contraceptives

impotence, nicotine and, 283

incontinence, anal sex and, 208–209

infidelity, 80–81, 93

inhibition in bed, alcohol use and, 293–294, 295–297, 301, 303; body image and, 11; masturbation and, 49; orgasm and, 39

inner lips. See labia minora

insecurities, body image and, 9–13

interfemoral sex, 223, 311

intimacy, 182, 207f

intrauterine device, 156–158, 157f. See also contraceptives

itching, gonorrhea, 94t; herpes, 104; human papilloma virus, 105t; parasitic STDs, 109–110; vaginosis, 98–99t

IUD, 156–158, 157f, 311. See also contraceptives

K

K-Y Jelly. See lubrication

Kegel exercises, 260–262, 263–266, 311

Kinsey Scale for Sexual Orientation, 64–65

kissing, as foreplay, 194

L

labia majora, description, 14f, 15, 17f, 311; during mutual masturbation, 221–223; oral sex and, 212–215

labia minora, description, 14f, 15, 17f, 311; doggie-style and, 206; during excitement stage, 25; masturbation and, 51–52, 221–223; oral sex and, 212–215

latex allergies, 139

latex condoms. See condoms

Liberator Shapes, 255. See also toys

lips, vaginal. See labia majora; labia minora

liquid X, 302. See also forced sex

lotion, body image and, 12–13

love, difficulties with, 75–76; expressing during foreplay, 198; vs. lust, 76–80; orgasm and, 34–35. See also relationships

loving your body, exercises, 11–12

lubrication, A-spot and, 233–234; anal sex and, 208, 209–210; gluteal sex and, 211; during a hand job, 219; masturbation and, 51, 53, 54; PC muscles and, 263; use of, 180; use with toys, 250; vaginal, 16; vaginosis and, 98

Lunelle, 161, 311. See also contraceptives

lust vs. love, 76–80. See also attraction

M

male sexual anatomy, 19–22, 19f, 21f

mammary glands, 16. See also breasts

man on top (position), 202–203. See also positions

marijuana, 284–285. See also drug use and sex

A POCKET SEXUALITY LIBRARY
Four illustrated, fun books *by* Richard Craze

pg. 1

THE POCKET BOOK OF SENSATIONAL ORGASMS

Designed for couples in loving relationships, this is a unique look at how couples can intensify, extend, and enhance orgasms.

Using techniques such as "The Tail of the Ostrich" and the "Two-Handed-Twist," partners can release inhibitions and share erotic adventures. The book also explains the difference between male and female orgasms; types of orgasms: vaginal, clitoral, G-spot, anal, multiple, mutual, and oral; and how to enhance sexual satisfaction with seduction and foreplay.

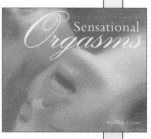

96 pages ... 64 color photos ... Paperback $11.95

THE POCKET BOOK OF FOREPLAY

Foreplay isn't just a prelude to the "real thing" — it's an experience to be enjoyed for itself. This book shows you how, with full-color pictures of the joys of foreplay, from "Setting the Scene" to "Reaching the Limits," and it's full of new foreplay ideas and even sexy Tantric techniques.

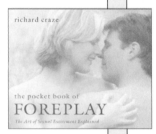

96 pages ... 68 color photos ... Paperback $10.95

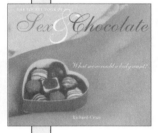

THE POCKET BOOK OF SEX AND CHOCOLATE

What more could a body want? Explore the pleasures of the ultimate combination — sex and chocolate. The suggestions for combining chocolate and sex range from saucy to classy. You learn about the best kinds of chocolate — and how to smear, lick, dribble, and, of course, eat it. Full of sensuous photographs, this book will give new meaning to the joy of chocolate.

96 pages ... 67 color photos ... Paperback $10.95

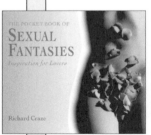

THE POCKET BOOK OF SEXUAL FANTASIES

Our imagination knows no bounds when it comes to sex and passion. This book explores how to get beyond inhibitions and act out fantasies. It guides you through the common kinds of fantasies — bondage, striptease, voyeurism, fetishism, toys, teasing, leather and lace, exhibitionism, and cross-dressing — and touches on how fantasy can become an art form or even a ritual.

96 pages ... 64 color photos ... Paperback $10.95

To order or for our FREE catalog or call (800) 266-5592

More Hunter House Books on
SEXUALITY & SENSUALITY

FEMALE EJACULATION & THE G-SPOT: Not Your Mother's Orgasm
Book *by* Deborah Sundahl; Foreworts by Annie Sprinkle and Alice Ladas

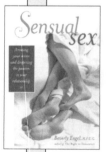

This open and down-to-earth book will help women reconnect with the G-spot and discover their natural ability to ejaculate. The approach respects women's doubts and fears, and invites those who are ready to connect with their power and desire to jump right in. Contents include: why some women ejaculate and others don't; exercises for strengthening and relaxing pelvic muscles; techniques, positions, and aids that help a woman ejaculate; men's role in helping their female partners to ejaculate.

Massage techniques and exercises to heal numbing in this sensitive area due to sexual trauma are also included.

240 pages ... 13 illus. ... Paperback $15.95

SEX TIPS & TALES FROM WOMEN WHO DARE: Exploring
the Exotic Erotic. *Edited by* Jo-Anne Baker. Contributors include Deborah Sundahl, Susie Bright, Annie Sprinkle, Joani Blank, Linda Montano, Jwala, Veronica Vera, Carol Queen, Kat Sunlove, Candida Royalle, Nan Kinney, and Nina Hartley.

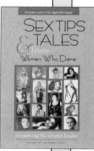

A remarkable collection of writings by women at the forefront of the sexual revolution. With credentials as varied as their backgrounds — from journalists and entrepreneurs to porn stars and transsexuals — they share intimate secrets on sex, self-love, and satisfaction. *Sex Tips & Tales from Women Who Dare* provides a stimulating perspective on sexuality as a life-long adventure.

"Dynamic and delicious..." — Eve Ensler, author of
The Vagina Monologues

256 pages. ... 30 b/w photos ... Paperback $13.95

SENSUAL SEX: Awakening Your Senses and Deepening
the Passion in Your Relationship *by* Beverly Engel, MFCC

Life is a sensual experience that we can smell, taste, touch — and enjoy. *Sensual Sex* brings that dimension to lovemaking. The one-of-a-kind "Reawakening Your Senses" program engages couples in a new level of physical exploration; "Deeper Love" offers an introduction to Tantric sexual ecstasy; and "The Four Seasons of Sensuous Passion" describes the stages of a long-term intimate relationship and sensual exercises that can strengthen each phase. Sensitively written and beautifully designed, this is a book to share, enjoy, and keep for a long time.

256 pages ... Paperback $14.95

Order online at www.hunterhouse.com ... all prices subject to change

EXTENDED MASSIVE ORGASM: How You Can Give and Receive
Intense Sexual Pleasure by Steve Bodansky, Ph.D., & Vera Bodansky, Ph.D.

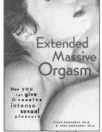

Yes, extended massive orgasms can be achieved! In this hands-on guide to doing it, Steve Bodansky and his wife, Vera, describe how to take the experience of sex to a new level of enjoyment.

The authors disclose stimulation techniques and uniquely sensitive areas known only to specialized researchers, recommend the best positions for orgasm, and offer strategic advice for every technique from seduction to kissing. With the help of this book you'll find it's never too late — or too early — to make your partner ecstatic in the bedroom.

224 pages ... 6 illus. ... 12 b/w photos ... Paperback $14.95

THE ILLUSTRATED GUIDE TO EXTENDED MASSIVE ORGASM
by Steve Bodansky, Ph.D., & Vera Bodansky, Ph.D.

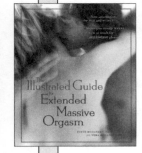

In this companion book, Steve and Vera Bodansky give much more detail about the best hand and body positions for performing and receiving EMO. More than 70 photographs and drawings illustrate genital anatomy and stimulation techniques, and the book covers new ground in the area of male arousal and orgasm.

Suddenly orgasm is no longer just a fleeting moment, but the beginning of lasting arousal that goes far beyond the bedroom.

256 pages ... 57 illus. ... 25 b/w photos ... Paperback $16.95

SIMULTANEOUS ORGASM and Other Joys of Sexual Intimacy
by Michael Riskin, Ph.D., & Anita Banker-Riskin, M.A.

Based on techniques developed at the Human Sexuality Institute, this guide shows couples how they can achieve the special, intimate experience of simultaneous orgasm. The book gives specific techniques and step-by-step instructions that help individuals achieve orgasm separately, and then simultaneously. Exercises include practical advice for relaxing and feeling comfortable with yourself and your partner. A separate section explains the purpose of the exercise and offers insights about how it can positively affect your relationship.

240 pages ... 9 b/w photos ... Paperback $14.95

To order or for our FREE catalog or call (800) 266-5592

ORDER FORM

10% DISCOUNT on orders of $50 or more —
20% DISCOUNT on orders of $150 or more —
30% DISCOUNT on orders of $500 or more —
On cost of books for fully prepaid orders

NAME

ADDRESS

CITY/STATE   ZIP/POSTCODE

PHONE   COUNTRY (outside of U.S.)

TITLE	QTY	PRICE	TOTAL
The Hot Guide to Safer Sex (paper)		@ $ 14.95	
Female Ejaculation & the G-Spot (paper)		@ $ 15.95	

Prices subject to change without notice

Please list other titles below:

		@ $	
		@ $	
		@ $	
		@ $	
		@ $	
		@ $	
		@ $	

Check here to receive our book catalog ☐   *FREE*

Shipping Costs
By Priority Mail: first book $4.50, each additional book $1.00
By UPS and to Canada: first book $5.50, each additional book $1.50
For rush orders and other countries call us at (510) 865-5282

TOTAL _____
Less discount @_____%   (_____)
TOTAL COST OF BOOKS _____
Calif. residents add sales tax _____
Shipping & handling _____
TOTAL ENCLOSED _____
Please pay in U.S. funds only

☐ Check   ☐ Visa   ☐ MasterCard   ☐ Discover

Card # _____ Exp. date _____

Signature _____

Complete and mail to:
Hunter House Inc., Publishers
PO Box 2914, Alameda CA 94501-0914
Website: www.hunterhouse.com
Orders: (800) 266-5592 or email: ordering@hunterhouse.com
Phone (510) 865-5282   Fax (510) 865-4295

HGS 6/2003